Case Studies in Anatomy

CASE STUDIES IN ANATOMY

SECOND EDITION

ERNEST LACHMAN, M.D.

Regents Professor of Anatomical and Radiological Sciences
University of Oklahoma School of Medicine

NEW YORK
OXFORD UNIVERSITY PRESS
LONDON TORONTO 1971

Sixth printing, 1978

Library of Congress Catalog Card Number: 71-140910
Printed in the United States of America

To my students,
past and present

Preface to Second Edition

Since the appearance of the first edition of this book, many changes have taken place in the educational program of American medical schools. Almost uniformly, the demand has been raised and met in the new curricula to expose the medical student from the beginning of his training to patient-oriented teaching programs. Thus the educational philosophy that was expressed in the preface to the first edition has been amply justified. More than ever, one of the primary reasons for study of the basic sciences in medical school is their application to the understanding and solving of problems in the clinical disciplines.

The second edition incorporates twelve additional case studies distributed over the various regions of the body. These have been published previously in *The New Physician*. They have been revised and amplified where necessary and their format adjusted to that of the previous case studies. All presentations have been reviewed and the terminology brought up to date. Many case studies have been enlarged with stress on conceptualizations and anatomical principles. Some cases have been thoroughly revised or re-written.

Warm thanks are again expressed to *The New Physician* and its editors for permission to utilize these case studies in this edition. The original work was, in part, supported by a grant from the National Fund for Medical Education.

Special appreciation is rendered to my friend and colleague, Dr. John E. Allison, for his fine drawings which illustrate the twelve additional cases. Most of these drawings are based on his own dissections.

Thanks are also due to my colleagues in the Department and a number of reviewers for their suggestions, which I have tried to incorporate in this presentation.

I am also most grateful to the Oxford University Press in New York and to their editors for their fine co-operation and their helpful suggestions.

Finally, I want to express my deep-felt thanks to our Departmental Secretary, Mrs. Pat Friedel, who again as in the first edition was most helpful and untiring in seeing this manuscript through to completion.

E. L.
Oklahoma City
November 1970

Preface to First Edition

In the teaching program in Gross Anatomy we face the well-known dilemma that at the time the student has to master a large body of anatomical information he is not aware of its application to clinical medicine. On the other hand when he is ready to utilize his knowledge at the bedside, he has forgotten a substantial part of this material. Yet the importance of anatomical reasoning and the application of anatomical principles in the explanation of clinical signs and events and in the design of therapeutic procedures can be exemplified almost from the first week of the basic course. This will strengthen the student's motivation for learning and satisfy his thirst for information relating to clinical medicine. We cannot afford to stifle this basic interest which has brought a large proportion of our students to medicine. The student can be made to realize from the beginning that his day-by-day learning is meaningful in terms of his future work as a physician.

Thus, the case studies presented in this book are directed specifically to the first and second year medical student for collateral reading either in the basic anatomy course or in advanced courses in the field. Elective courses in the clinical years can readily be based on the exercises presented here, particularly if they are supplemented by pertinent and specialized dissections, executed by the student himself. Residents may find these case reports useful in their review studies, particularly for board examinations.

In each case a short history, physical findings, diagnosis, therapy, and further course are given. This is followed by a discussion of the material from the anatomical viewpoint, generally in the form of questions posed and answers given. The underlying anatomy is illustrated by drawings. This presentation lends itself to self-study since all questions formulated are answered in detail and in a comprehensive discussion of the subject matter.

The individual exercises are based on case histories chosen from the literature and from the author's experience and present a composite picture that exemplifies the characteristic anatomical features of the problem under discussion. In a few instances the history is taken from one of the classical collections of masterfully composed case studies available in the literature, such as the works of Hertzler, Cabot, or Kanavel. This type of presentation should call the student's attention to a stimulating form of medical instruction. In this connection it may be worth noting that in law classes in American universities the case method has been utilized for many years, even in the freshman year, whereby principles of law are illustrated by actual cases and real-life legal problems.

All case histories contained in this book have appeared previously in *The New Physician,* but in many instances their format has been changed, a large number have been revised and amplified.

Grateful acknowledgement is made to *The New Physician* and its editorial staff for permission to utilize these case histories.

Permission was also granted by the C. V. Mosby Company to use part of two case histories from Hertzler's *Clinical Surgery by Case Histories;* by the W. B. Saunders Company to utilize a portion of one case history published in Volume I of Cabot's *Differential Diagnosis;* by Lea and Febiger to use a case history from Kanavel's *Infections of the Hands;* by Doctors R. D. Duncan and M. E. Myers, Dr. L. B. Rose, and Dr. D. H. O'Donoghue to utilize material from individual case histories published by them. To these publishers and authors I express my grateful appreciation.

Thanks are due to the artists Mr. E. F. Hiser and Dr. J. E. Allison for their fine co-operation in executing the drawings, and to Frank Romano.

I am greatly indebted to Doctors G. H. Daron and K. K. Faulkner for many thoughtful suggestions.

Especially warm thanks are rendered to Mrs. Pat Friedel, our department secretary, whose tireless efforts were so helpful in bringing the work to speedy completion.

E. L.
Oklahoma City
October 1964

Contents

Head and Neck

1 Facial Paralysis

A 36-year-old woman librarian slept close to an open window on a cold drafty night. She woke up in the morning with some aching pain in and around the ear; the right side of her face felt numb and swollen. On arising she noticed that her face was distorted and deformed. She could not close her right eye completely. She had some difficulty in speaking, eating, and drinking. Food seemed to collect between her teeth and her right cheek. Saliva and liquids that she tried to drink ran out of the right corner of her mouth, although she had no difficulty swallowing. She became quite apprehensive and consulted a physician.

EXAMINATION

On examination the right side of the face of the patient appears immobile and without expression. All wrinkles have disappeared from her right forehead; the right nasolabial fold is less distinct than the left. The right eyebrow droops and there is sagging of the right lower eyelid. There is some flow of tears down the side of her face. The nose and mouth seem deviated toward the unaffected side and the right corner of her mouth is sagging.

On further examination the following facial movements prove to be interfered with. The patient cannot frown on the right side when asked to do so. When patient attempts to shut her eyes, the right eye does not close completely. She cannot purse her lips tightly, whistle, or puff out her cheeks. Asked to show her teeth, she uncovers them only on her unaffected left side and her lips seem to be drawn to the left side. On attempt at laughing, the distortion of her face becomes considerably more noticeable and disfiguring.

DIAGNOSIS

All signs and symptoms of this patient point to a disease known as facial paralysis or Bell's palsy, the latter term perpetuating the name and memory of Charles Bell, a British anatomist and surgeon who first described the disease in 1821.

THERAPY AND FURTHER COURSE

Under treatment with analgesics and local heat, the pain disappeared. Later, electric stimulation of the involved muscles, massage, and active exercises were resorted to. After five weeks the patient was almost completely recovered and only traces of the previous paralysis, particularly around the mouth, could be demonstrated.

DISCUSSION

The exact cause of the condition is not known, but the paralysis of the facial nerve is presumed to be due to an inflammation of the facial nerve in the facial canal. Remember the course of the facial nerve in the petrous portion of the temporal bone where even slight swelling of the nerve within its tight-fitting bony surroundings would subject the nerve to destructive pressure. What is the name of the foramen at the lower end of the canal, through which the nerve emerges from the skull? Is this also the site of entrance of an artery that supplies the facial nerve within the canal? Some authors ascribe the damage of the nerve to constriction of this artery caused by chilling. Of what artery is it most commonly a branch? The facial nerve emerges from the skull through the stylomastoid foramen. This is the site of entrance of the stylomastoid artery, a branch of the posterior auricular artery of the external carotid artery.

Effects of paralysis on facial muscles

The motor deficiencies present in this case exemplify the actions of the facial muscles innervated by the seventh nerve. These muscles are conventionally grouped under the heading of mimetic muscles or muscles of facial expression and are responsible for voluntary movements of the face and emotional expression. How do you explain the disappearance of wrinkles of the forehead and certain facial folds in facial paralysis? It must be realized that some folds of the skin are brought about by habitual wrinkling of the skin, as on the forehead in frowning and around the eyes in squinting. With paralysis of the facial muscles, such as the frontalis which normally is responsible for transverse folds on the forehead, or the orbicularis oculi which causes "crow's feet," the tonus of these muscles, which attach in part to the skin, is lost and the folds disappear.

Paralysis of what muscle explains the inability to close the right eye and causes the sagging of the lower eyelid? The former deficiency leads to the most serious complication of facial paralysis, that is, inflammation of the conjunctiva and cornea, and possible corneal ulceration. The sagging of the lower lid results in its eversion and the spilling of tears, as in this case. Where do tears normally drain? What muscle opens the eye? Is it affected in facial palsy? The muscle whose paralysis is responsible for sometimes serious eye complications is the orbicularis oculi which when functioning acts like a windshield wiper to keep the cornea moist and clean. Tears normally drain through the lacrimal puncta and canaliculi into the lacrimal sac and from there via the nasolacrimal duct into the nose. The muscle responsible for opening the eye is the levator palpebrae superioris, which is supplied by the unaffected oculomotor nerve.

Paralysis of which important muscle causes food to collect between cheek and teeth and is responsible for the inability to whistle? The buccinator has the essential function of maintaining tension of the cheek and to keep food from passing between cheek and teeth. It also prevents the mucous membrane of the cheek from being caught between the teeth in the act of mastication.

The inability to purse the lips and show the teeth of the affected side is due to paralysis of the orbicularis oris, which through its action as a whole or in parts can either protrude the lips as in pouting or draw them against the teeth.

The absence of the mimic expression of smile and laughter is the resultant of the dysfunction of numerous small facial muscles, such as the zygomaticus, the risorius, the nasalis, and the levator labii superioris, all of which have in common a superficial subcutaneous location, the absence of a muscle fascia, and insertion into the skin. Their paralysis is responsible for the previously mentioned characteristic feature of Bell's palsy: loss, on the paralyzed side, of expression of emotion, such as surprise and attention, joy and sorrow.

Involvement of the scalp muscles (frontalis and occipitalis) and the extrinsic muscles of the ear as well as of the stylohyoid and posterior belly of the digastric muscle is difficult to demonstrate.

Ear symptoms and taste deficiency in facial paralysis

Occasionally, the stapedius muscle also is paralyzed. Would that give any clue as to the site of attack of the noxious agent? This paralysis can only occur if the facial nerve is affected in the facial canal, central to the origin of its branch to the stapedius muscle. Since it is the function of the stapedius muscle to dampen the vibrations of the ossicles by tilting the footplate of the stapes, what is the result of paralysis of this muscle? The consequent increased acuity of the sense of hearing may be quite annoying to the patient.

How do you account for the aching pain in and around the ear and the sensation of numbness in the face? Does the facial nerve contain any general somatic afferent fibers? In which ganglion are their cell bodies located? The geniculate ganglion contains the cell bodies of these somatic sensory fibers. The peripheral course of the fibers mediating pain from the ear in facial palsy is somewhat uncertain. Two pathways are possible: one by way of a communication from the facial nerve in the lowest part of the facial canal to the auricular branch of the vagus and with it to the external ear; the other accompanying the motor fibers of the posterior auricular branch of the facial nerve. Whether the facial nerve contains fibers mediating deep sensibility of the face including deep-seated pain is disputed.

Absence of clinically demonstrable signs of involvement of the chorda tympani does not help in locating the site of the lesion below the origin of this nerve since visceral efferent impulses as well as visceral afferent impulses, which ordinarily utilize the chorda tympani, may also follow other pathways. This makes it frequently impossible to demonstrate deficiencies in case of damage of the chorda tympani. Where would interruption of taste be noticeable if the chorda tympani were involved and no alternate path for taste impulses were available? Taste would be interrupted in the anterior two-thirds of the tongue on the affected side.

2 Trigeminal Neuralgia

A 60-year-old housewife has suffered from attacks of severe, sharp, stabbing pain in the right lower eyelid, on the right side of her nose and cheek, and the right upper lip for more than one year. These paroxysms of pain last only a few seconds, but seem to the patient so unbearable that she requests immediate help. She reports that when the pain started it was less intense, occurred less often, and was felt only at the site of the nose, rather than in the larger area where it is now located. She also states that the pain ceased for a period of four months, but then returned in greater intensity and frequency. She had several teeth extracted in the upper jaw and underwent drainage of the maxillary sinus, without relief. Chewing, drinking, washing, drying her face, or blowing her nose bring on these attacks. A light touch to the side of the nose likewise precipitates a paroxysm of pain. The patient protects her face against touch and cold drafts with a shawl. On questioning, she states that the pain is always confined to her right side and never crosses the midline.

EXAMINATION

During the examination an attack is observed in which the patient winces and contorts her face in a tic-like fashion. Due to her difficulties in eating and drinking, she has lost fifteen pounds and appears dehydrated. On neurological examination no motor defects or interference with any modality of sensation conducted by the trigeminal nerve can be discovered. Examination of the function of the other cranial nerves is also negative. Except for the patient appearing anxious and tense, the physical examination is non-contributory.

DIAGNOSIS

Neuralgia (tic douloureux) of the maxillary division of the trigeminal nerve.

THERAPY AND FURTHER COURSE

The patient was given tranquilizers and analgesics. In addition, several medications were tried which are said to be specific for the treatment of trigeminal neuralgia. These included antiepileptic drugs and injections of Vitamin B_1 and B_{12}. She was seen regularly, but the treatment gave her only temporary relief. Since the pain continued unabated, she requested surgical measures. Under local anesthesia, 1 cc. of 95 per cent alcohol was injected into the maxillary division of the trigeminal nerve within the pterygopalatine fossa just beyond the exit of the nerve from the foramen rotundum.

For the next fifteen months the patient had complete relief from the attacks of pain. She gained considerable weight and was quite comfortable, but complained of annoying numbness and paresthesias (tingling and burning) in the area supplied by the maxillary nerve (Fig. 1A and B).

One and a half years after the alcohol injection into the maxillary nerve she again began to suffer attacks of excruciating pain. The maxillary nerve was blocked for the second time with an alcohol injection in the pterygopalatine fossa, and this time the pain-free period lasted only about eight months. Consequently, a more radical approach was decided upon, i.e. the cutting of the sensory root of the trigeminal nerve posterior to the trigeminal ganglion (rhizotomy).

A temporal extradural approach to the sensory root of the trigeminal nerve was chosen. The patient was put in a sitting position in a chair, akin to a dental chair, with the head held

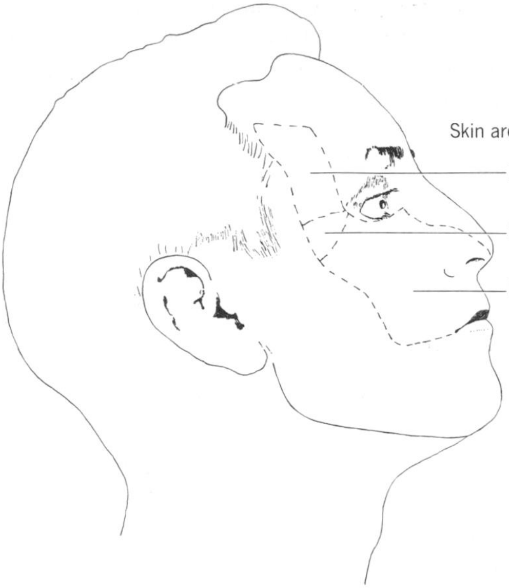

Figure 1A demonstrates skin areas supplied by maxillary division of trigeminal nerve.

upright. General anesthesia was applied intratracheally. A vertical incision was made in front of the external auditory meatus and was extended upward from the zygoma. The temporal fascia and the underlying temporalis muscle were split and retracted. With a burr, an opening was drilled through the squama of the temporal bone and enlarged to 4 cm in diameter. By blunt dissection the dura was stripped from the anterior slope of the petrous bone and the floor of the middle cranial fossa, and the middle meningeal artery was located at the foramen spinosum, cut, coagulated, and ligated. Further stripping of the dura uncovered the mandibular division of the trigeminal nerve at the site where it enters the foramen ovale just medial to and in front of the foramen spinosum. Following the posterior border of the mandibular nerve (V-3) the surgeon was led to the trigeminal (gasserian) ganglion and from there in a posteromedial and upward direc-

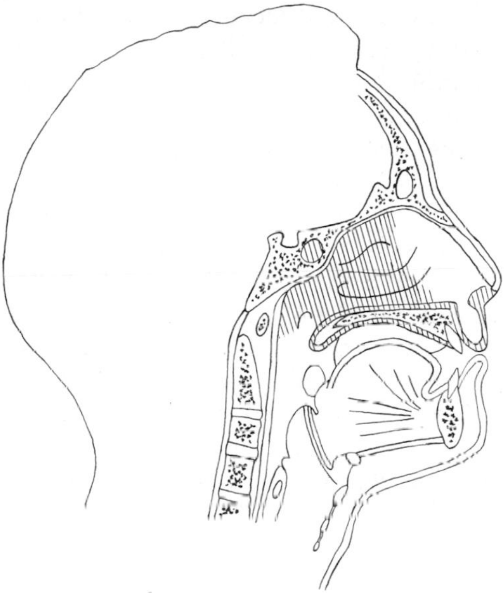

Figure 1B demonstrates mucosal areas supplied by maxillary division of trigeminal nerve. Keep in mind that areas of anesthesia after injection or surgical intervention are somewhat smaller due to overlap by other divisions of the trigeminal and other cranial and cervical nerves.

tion to its sensory root. This root was uncovered by incision into the dural/arachnoidal sleeve of the ganglion and root. The subarachnoid space around these structures was opened, a procedure that resulted in a flow of cerebrospinal fluid. This was aspirated until the field was dry. Since it was the intent of the surgeon to sever only the sensory root fibers from the second and third division of the trigeminal nerve, but not the first, and since these occupy a fairly well defined position within the lateral part of the root, a subtotal section of the root was possible. This section was undertaken about one-half centimeter posterior to the ganglion and did not include the sensory fibers of the ophthalmic division or the motor root of the third division (Fig. 2). The sensory fibers of the ophthalmic nerve occupy a superomedial location within the sensory root of the trigeminal nerve. Occasionally, they are separated from the fibers of the other two divisions by a cleft, which of course makes selective section easier. The motor root of cranial V can be identified by its somewhat more opaque appearance, by its direction, and especially by its position deep to the sensory root, with the motor root running obliquely downward and forward to join the sensory part of the mandibular division at the foramen ovale. After all bleeding points had been controlled, the incision was closed by approximating and suturing the cut ends of the temporal muscle, temporal fascia, and skin. The patient recovered speedily from the operation and was free of pain. Her only complaint was numbness of the right side of her face. From previous alcohol injections, the patient was familiar with these side effects and tolerated them well.

DISCUSSION

General definition of trigeminal neuralgia

This patient suffered from trigeminal neuralgia involving the maxillary (second) division of the trigeminal nerve. It was temporarily relieved by alcohol injection into the nerve and cured by subtotal retrogasserian neurotomy (rhizotomy). The patient was typical as far as age, sex, and involved division of the trigeminal nerve is concerned, the disease being more common in the elderly female and the maxillary division of the trigeminal nerve. Some authors designate the mandibular division as the one most frequently involved.

Although not fatal, trigeminal neuralgia represents one of the most catastrophic afflictions of man, which may drive the sufferer to suicide.

The neuralgia consists of paroxysmal attacks of pain which involve the area of the sensory distribution of one or more divisions of the trigeminal nerve. The attacks are characterized by their short duration, by intervals of relief from pain, by their unilaterality, by the absence of objective neurological findings, either on clinical examination or at autopsy, and by the frequent presence of trigger zones in the face or the mucosa. These zones, when lightly touched, may induce an attack. While in a limited number of cases infections and neoplasms as well as toxic, vascular, or nutritive factors may play a role in bringing about this condition, in most instances no cause can be found. As in our patient, there is no involvement of the paranasal sinuses and extraction of teeth does not bring any relief.

The term "tic douloureux" is somewhat misleading in that it might be deduced that a muscular spasm is the cause of the pain. Actually the sequence is reversed, since it is the excruciating pain that causes the patient to wince and grimace by contorting his facial muscles.

Course and distribution of the maxillary nerve and the applied anatomy of maxillary nerve block

The only division involved in our case is the maxillary division (V-2) of the trigeminal nerve. What is its course to its peripheral area of distribution and what regions of skin and mucosa does it supply? The maxillary nerve, as this division also is frequently called, runs from the middle portion of the trigeminal ganglion along the lateral wall of the cavernous sinus and leaves the middle cranial fossa through the foramen rotundum to enter the pterygopalatine fossa. Here it can be reached by alcohol injection as was done in our case (Fig. 2). Inspection of a skull demonstrates that the injection needle has to be inserted in the infratemporal fossa below the zygomatic arch and in front of the ramus of the mandible to pass through the pterygopalatine fissure into the pterygopalatine fossa. Here it reaches the maxillary nerve just after the latter leaves the foramen rotundum and before it has divided into its branches of distribution.

What regions of skin and mucosa are supplied by branches of the maxillary nerve? The skin over the anterior part of the temples and part of the cheek are innervated by the zygomatic nerve, one of the smaller terminal branches of the maxillary nerve. The main branch of the maxillary nerve, the infraorbital,

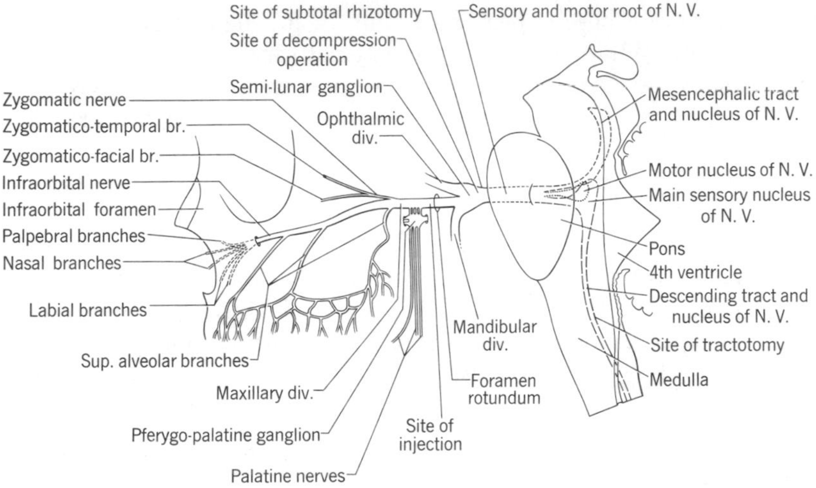

Figure 2 depicts trigeminal nuclei and tracts, root, ganglion, and divisions of trigeminal nerve and distribution area of maxillary division. Notice the sites of surgical intervention, i.e., tractotomy, rhizotomy, decompression, and alcohol injection.

enters the orbit through the infraorbital fissure, passes along the infraorbital groove and canal, and emerges on the face through the infraorbital foramen to supply the skin of the lower eyelid, the lateral side of the nose, and the upper lip. Other branches, either of the maxillary or the infraorbital nerve, supply the mucous membrane of the paranasal sinuses, the nasopharynx, the palatine tonsil, the soft palate, the teeth and gums of the upper jaw, the inside of the nasal cavity, the conjunctiva of the lower eyelid, and the mucous membrane of the upper lip (Figs. 1A, B, and 2)

The sites mentioned define the location of the excruciating pain in neuralgia of this division, although the pain may be confined to smaller areas of skin or mucosa, such as the infraorbital region or parts of the palate. We also understand why in neuralgia of this division the upper teeth are so often extracted and the paranasal sinuses drained, as was the case with our patient, unfortunately with the expected negative result.

The area of anesthesia after alcohol injection into the maxillary nerve roughly coincides with the anatomical distribution of its branches, although allowance must be made for some overlap in the sensory supply of skin and mucosa from other divisions of the trigeminal nerve and from other cranial and cervical nerves. As a result of the anesthesia after blocking of the maxillary nerve or sectioning of its root the patient often complains of disturbing numbness in the denervated area.

How do you explain the frequent recurrence of the neuralgic pain after alcohol injection into the nerve, as happened in our patient? While the alcohol injection leads to disintegration of the sensory nerve fibers and therefore to interruption of pain transmission, the relief is generally only temporary, since nerve fibers regenerate from their proximal ends above the line of injection. Recurring injections become less and less successful since the scarring and fibrosis in the nerve prevent the alcohol from reaching all fibers.

Applied anatomy of gasserian ganglion injection

The pitfall of regeneration of the sensory fibers and recurrence of neuralgia is avoided by alcohol injection into the ganglion itself, because here the injection destroys the cell bodies of the sensory fibers which then cannot regenerate. However, this procedure has fallen into disfavor due to the dangers and complications connected with it.

The possible harmful effects of trigeminal ganglion destruction by injection can be understood by familiarity with its anatomy. The trigeminal (semilunar or gasserian) ganglion is the equivalent of a dorsal root ganglion of a spinal nerve and contains pseudounipolar cell bodies. These send out T-shaped processes that divide into a central fiber (axon) which runs in the sensory root of the trigeminal nerve to the brain stem, and a peripheral fiber (dendrite) which conducts sensory impulses from the periphery to the ganglion cell. The trigeminal ganglion lies in a slight depression in the apex of the petrous portion of the temporal bone within the middle cranial fossa. The ganglion is surrounded by a sleeve of dura/arachnoid, which is a diverticular extension of the meninges of the posterior cranial fossa. The meninges and subarachnoid space extend over the posterior portion of the ganglion where they fuse with the connective tissue around the ganglion, thus obliterating the extension of the subarachnoid space. The danger of injection of the ganglion lies in its described close relation to the subarachnoid space. Customarily, the ganglion is injected through the foramen ovale. If the needle penetrates too deeply, it enters the subarachnoid space and the alcohol may be injected into the cerebrospinal fluid. It then "passes to the base of the brain, causing a dreadful series of paralyses of all the nerves on the side of the injection, in addition to pronounced disturbance of the cerebellum" (Dandy). The nerves involved are cranial III, IV, VI, VII, VIII, and possibly other cranial nerves. Paralysis of the ocular and facial muscles and diminution or loss of hearing is the end result. These effects may be permanent. Other dangers are based on the close relationship of the ganglion to the cavernous sinus and the internal carotid artery within it. Thus, the injecting needle may perforate the sinus and enter the internal carotid artery. The danger to the motor portion of the trigeminal nerve and the complication of keratitis through ganglion injection will be discussed in conjunction with sectioning of the sensory root.

Subtotal retrogasserian neurotomy

As has been stated before, after failure of alcohol injections into the involved division, the treatment of choice is subtotal retrogasserian neurotomy by way of a temporal approach (Fig. 2). The operation has been described. The mortality rate is around 1 per cent and less in the hands of experienced neurosurgeons. Subtotal in contrast to complete section of the sensory root is possible by virtue of the fact that the fibers in the sensory root posterior to the ganglion are still arranged according to the three divisions of the nerve, with the fibers from the ophthalmic division lying more medial and superior, while those of the maxillary and mandibular divisions are located more lateral and inferior. Why did the surgeon in our case not just sever the fibers coming from the maxillary division, since these were the only ones involved, rather than include the mandibular fibers? The maxillary and mandibular components are not as easily separated from each other as they are from the ophthalmic. A second important reason is the frequent spread of trigeminal neuralgia from the second to the third division and vice versa, with the ophthalmic division being only rarely involved. Such spread would necessitate a second intracranial operation, which is thus avoided. It is most important to preserve the fibers coming from the ophthalmic division, if at all possible, because destruction of the sensory fibers from the cornea leads to abolishment of the protective corneal reflex. The absence of this reflex makes the cornea susceptible to inflammation and ulceration due to desiccation and trauma. A serious keratitis and possible loss of eyesight on this side may follow denervation of the first division.

The other portion of the trigeminal nerve to be spared is the motor root which is not too difficult to separate from the sensory root. The minor portion of the trigeminal nerve, as the motor root is frequently called, runs along the undersurface of the major portion from medial to lateral, to join the mandibular branch with which it passes through the foramen ovale. Why would inadvertent destruction of the motor root usually result only in temporary paralysis, and what muscles would be involved? The muscles temporarily paralyzed would be the muscles of mastication on one side. The destruction generally would not be permanent because section of the minor portion severs only the peripheral portion of the axons. The cell bodies within their nucleus in the pons (motor nucleus) and the proximal part of the axons remain intact and allow the axons to regenerate (Fig. 2). Are the fibers in the motor root of the trigeminal nerve exclusively motor, as the designation might indicate? The motor root also contains sensory fibers from the mesencephalic nucleus of the trigeminal nerve (Fig. 2). These are proprioceptive and join the motor fibers to supply the same muscles with afferent fibers.

Interruption of the middle meningeal artery

In the description of the surgical procedure used in our patient it was mentioned that after stripping of the dura from the middle cranial fossa, the meningeal artery was cut and coagulated. Coagulation at the site of section protects against the risk of future extradural hemorrhage, which is a rather rare complication of this procedure. Where does the middle meningeal artery come from and how does it enter the skull? What does the artery supply and how well is its interruption tolerated? The middle meningeal artery is a branch of the first division of the maxillary artery of the external carotid and enters the skull through the foramen spinosum. It is a major source of blood supply to the adjacent skull bones in addition to providing for the dura mater. After ligation of the middle meningeal artery, meningeal branches from other sources assume the distribution of arterial blood to the areas previously supplied by the middle meningeal artery.

Complication of facial paralysis

Posterior rhizotomy may not infrequently result in facial paralysis, a complication which fortunately is only temporary (lasting up to six months). Although the explanation for this complication is not quite clear, most authors ascribe it to traction on the greater superficial petrosal nerve at surgery. It will be remembered that the greater superficial petrosal nerve branches off the facial nerve at the geniculate ganglion to emerge from the anterior slope of the petrous bone just lateral to the trigeminal ganglion and then courses beneath the ganglion. If the dura is stripped from the skull at this point, the nerve may be stretched and injured, resulting in edema which spreads to and compresses the facial nerve at the site of the geniculate ganglion.

The anatomy of recurrence of neuralgia

In evaluating the success of retrogasserian neurotomy, it cannot be overlooked that the operation is not always successful and that the paroxysmal attacks continue or recur later. This has been ascribed to the possibility that some sensory ganglion cells might be located outside the ganglion itself along the posterior root, proximal to the point of section. However, if the section severs all centrally directed fibers from the involved division beyond their cell bodies, regeneration of the fibers from the ganglion, even if it occurs, stops short of the pons. None of the regenerating fibers can penetrate the pia-glial barrier to establish central connections which are essential for the return of the paroxysmal attacks.

Physiology of paresthesias

The main complication of trigeminal root section, however, is the presence not only of numbness, which is unavoidable and well tolerated by the great majority of patients, but of paresthesias such as creeping sensations, burning, and itching. About 10 per cent of operated patients are severely disturbed by this effect, which is not paroxysmal as the original neuralgia, but is continuous and unremitting (anesthesia dolorosa). Some patients have declared that they are unhappier after the surgery than before. The cause of these paresthesias is difficult to establish. One might postulate that the absence of sensory input from the periphery after rhizotomy might disturb the balance of perception so that peripheral stimuli arising from the neighboring area via sensory fibers from other cranial nerves such as cranial VII, IX, and X, and cervical II and III, might evoke increased responses from the sensory and spinal nuclei of the trigeminal nerve.

Tractotomy of the spinal tract of nerve V

This brings us to a discussion of a newer and theoretically very appealing surgical approach to the treatment of trigeminal neuralgia, i.e. the section of the descending or spinal tract of the trigeminal nerve in the medulla. This operation (tractotomy) aims at interruption of all pain pathways in the trigeminal nerve with preservation of most of the touch sensation and avoidance of numbness and objectionable paresthesias (Fig. 2). However, the approach is considerably more complex and hazardous than subtotal rhizotomy and may not produce the desired results of complete analgesia. Lately due to its risk, complications, and ineffectiveness in a number of cases, the value of tractotomy has become quite doubtful.

Decompression operation

Two new approaches are still under investigation, but deserve attention. One is based on the not yet proved assumption that trigeminal neuralgia may be due to compression of its root and ganglion at the apex of the petrous bone. The operation consequently consists of simply opening the dural envelope over the ganglion and adjacent posterior root where the latter passes over the superior ridge of the petrous bone. A considerable number of patients have obtained relief from this operation, but the recurrence rate is rather high and there is frequently damage to other adjacent cranial nerves, particularly those controlling eye movements.

The surgery of intentional slight trauma to the ganglion

A different interpretation of the favorable results of the decompression operation, i.e. that the relief is due to slight compression and damage to the ganglion itself and the adjacent root, has induced other neurosurgeons to compress and slightly traumatize the ganglion and posterior root intentionally. Good results with absence of pain and no significant loss of other modalities of sensation have been observed.

Thus, trigeminal neuralgia, although its cause is still obscure, is being attacked surgically with good results.

3 Cavernous Sinus Thrombosis

A 32-year-old business executive returns from a hunting trip, where living conditions had been rather primitive, with high fever and severe headaches and in a generally bad state of health. He relates that about six days earlier he developed a boil on the right upper lip which resulted from a cut while shaving. He concedes that he had squeezed the boil. He is seen by his family physician who gives him penicillin injections and keeps him under close observation. Since the patient does not improve, but becomes very restless and rather delirious, he is transferred the same day to the hospital.

On admission the patient is found to be acutely ill with septic temperatures and frequent chills. He vomits at intervals, and from time to time becomes delirious. In his clearer moments he complains of nausea and severe headache, particularly on the right side.

EXAMINATION

On examination the patient shows rigidity of his neck muscles and various other clinical signs of meningeal irritation. His upper lip is hard and markedly swollen to about twice its normal size and is dusky red. There are some darkly colored crusts covering the right side of the upper lip, with some oozing of pus from several points. The right cheek and right side of his nose are swollen and hard to the touch. The right upper and lower eyelids are swollen as are the palpebral and bulbar conjunctivae. The right eyeball protrudes farther forward than the left (exophthalmos). Examination of the right eye is made difficult by the temporarily delirious state of the patient and the swelling of the eyelids. The fundus of the right eye shows dilation and engorgement of the retinal veins, and some edema of the optic nerve at the papilla. All voluntary movements of the right ocular muscles are abolished. This also includes the superior oblique and lateral rectus muscles. In his more lucid moments the patient complains of severe pain in his right eye. His vision in this eye is severely impaired. He also notices tingling and burning (paresthesia) at the right forehead, the right side of his nose, and the upper portion of his face. There seems to be some hardening along the course of the right facial vein.

On later examination he also shows some swelling of the left eyelid with some protrusion of the left eyeball and inability to abduct the left eye completely. Repeated blood cultures are positive for *Staphylococcus aureus.* The patient has marked leukocytosis and his differential blood count also indicates the presence of an acute infection.

DIAGNOSIS

Deep-seated staphylococcic infection of the subcutaneous tissue of the upper lip (carbuncle), infectious cavernous sinus thrombosis on the right and beginning cavernous sinus thrombosis on the left, with right-sided paralysis of all ocular muscles (ophthalmoplegia) and abducens paralysis on the left. Staphylococcic septicemia.

THERAPY

The patient is immediately put on intravenous antibiotics which include large doses of penicillin, sulfadiazine, and broad spectrum antibiotics. Local warm, moist dressings are applied to both eyes and the right side of his face. Narcotics are given to stop the pain.

FURTHER COURSE

The patient responds only slowly to the antibiotic treatment. His septic temperatures and severe illness persist for several days and only gradually subside. There is some sloughing of the subcutaneous tissue of the upper lip. Ocular function improves only gradually, but finally returns to normal. Antibiotic treatment is continued for approximately two weeks. The patient is discharged after three weeks, having made a complete recovery.

DISCUSSION

We are dealing here with infectious cavernous sinus thrombosis, a condition which before the advent of antibiotic treatment was almost invariably fatal. Where did the infection start? The infection began as an innocuous-appearing boil in the hair follicles of the upper lip, a rather common occurrence. How did it spread to the cavernous sinus? There is a rich venous plexus of labial veins to the outside of the main muscle mass of the lips, the orbicularis oris. Squeezing of the boil by the patient and the never-ceasing motion of the labial muscles which are traversed by numerous veins led to propagation of infected material, first in the finer venules, then in the smaller and larger veins draining the lips, with resulting infectious thrombosis of these veins (thrombophlebitis).

Facial vein, its tributaries and communications

Into what vein do the labial veins drain? The labial veins are tributaries of the facial vein, which usually terminates in the internal jugular vein or more rarely in the external jugular vein. Was the facial vein involved in our case? What is its course in the face? The facial vein was thrombosed and could be felt as a hardened cord. It runs posterolateral to the facial artery in front of the masseter muscle where it passes across the mandible. More important for the spread of the disease is the communication of the beginning of the facial vein, the angular

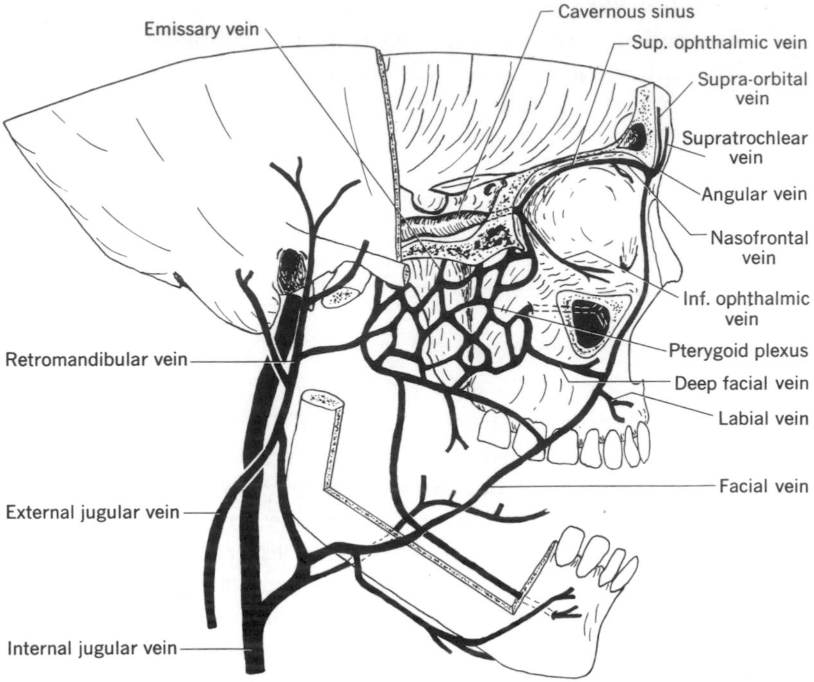

Figure 1 shows the communications of the facial vein and pterygoid plexus with the cavernous sinus.

vein, with the superior ophthalmic vein, and through it with the cavernous sinus (Fig. 1). Either the infection spreads discontinuously by means of an embolus (detached clot) from the face via the facial and angular veins and through the superior ophthalmic vein into the cavernous sinus, or there is an infectious thrombosis extending by continuity through the same vascular channels. The end result is a septic thrombosis of the cavernous sinus.

Is there an anatomical feature that facilitates the spread of infection to the cavernous sinus? The absence of valves in the veins of the face makes it possible for the venous blood to flow in either direction, toward the neck and the internal jugular vein or in the opposite direction toward the beginning of the facial vein at the inner angle of the eye. How is the angular vein at this site formed? The supratrochlear and supraorbital veins cross the forehead to unite at the upper medial corner of the orbit to form the angular vein, which then continues across the face as the facial vein, receiving tributaries from the eyelids, the side of the nose, and the lips. It is the important communication of the angular vein with the superior ophthalmic vein, often called the nasofrontal vein, that is responsible for the serious prognosis of infection in the area drained by the facial vein (Fig. 1).

Are there fascial layers surrounding the facial muscles which might limit the spread of infection? The muscles of facial expression are located in the subcutaneous tissue and are intimately connected with the skin. Since they are lacking fascial septa, no barrier stands in the way of propagation of infection. On the contrary, as has been mentioned, the contraction of these muscles, as in speaking or eating, tends to milk infectious material along the venous channels. Narcotics to quiet the patient and a liquid diet are, therefore, part of the therapy.

Is ligation of the angular vein, which was once used as a therapeutic measure, a rational procedure for the prevention of spread of the infection, or are there other venous channels to the cavernous sinus that could bypass the ligated vein? The latter is the case. There is a large communication from the facial vein via the deep facial vein to the pterygoid plexus. The latter anastomoses with the cavernous sinus by means of emissary veins that pass through foramina in the base of the skull. Ligation of the angular vein is therefore fruitless.

Are other surgical interventions such as opening of the carbuncle on the upper lip indicated? Cutting through infected tissues may spread the infection and generally results in worsening of the condition.

Are there other areas in the face besides the upper lip from which the infection could be propagated to the cavernous sinus? Any portion of the skin of the face which is drained by the facial vein can serve as the site of a primary focus. Boils of the nasal cavity, of the cheeks, eyelids, eyebrows, forehead, and lower lip, all have on occasion been the source of this dangerous complication, the commonest cause being a nasal furuncle.

Emissary veins

Could deeper regions of the head be the primary site of infection that is transmitted via venous channels to the cavernous sinus? Anatomically formulated, the question is: What veins besides the facial establish communications with the cavernous sinus and can serve as a pathway for the spread of infectious material to the sinus? The pharyngeal and pterygoid plexuses communicate with the cavernous sinus by way of emissary veins that pass through the foramen ovale and adjacent foramina. The pterygoid plexus also anastomoses with the inferior ophthalmic vein by a vein traversing the inferior orbital fissure, the inferior ophthalmic vein being a direct or indirect tributary of the cavernous sinus (Fig. 1). All the aforementioned veins, as well as the previously discussed superior ophthalmic vein, drain important regions of the head that frequently harbor infection. Thus, we understand that tonsillar and paratonsillar abscesses, dental infections, particularly after extractions, infections of the paranasal sinuses and the orbit, and posttraumatic infections of the face, the maxilla, or frontal bone all may lead to infectious cavernous sinus thrombosis.

What is the definition of an emissary vein? Can the ophthalmic veins be regarded as emissary veins? What is the direction of blood flow in emissary veins? Emissary veins are communications between intracranial venous sinuses and extracranial veins. They are thin-walled, valveless vessels that pass through cranial openings. Blood in them may flow in either direction. Their presence represents a safety mechanism which comes into play when there is an increase in intracranial venous pressure that might otherwise endanger the brain. On the other hand, the blood flow may be reversed, going from the outside to the sinuses, if there is an obstruction in the extracranial veins as in our case of thrombosis of the facial vein. In the sense that the ophthalmic veins establish a communication between the facial veins and the cavernous sinus, they can be regarded as emissary veins. Again, the blood flow in them can be in either direction, toward the cavernous sinus or toward the facial veins, depending on the ever-changing venous pressure conditions.

Cavernous sinus

The superior ophthalmic vein is the main tributary of the cavernous sinus. It enters the sinus at the superior orbital fissure. How does the cavernous sinus drain? It is continuous posteriorly at the apex of the petrous bone with, and drains its blood into the superior and inferior petrosal sinuses and through them into the transverse sinus and the internal jugular vein. Retrograde spread of infection from the ear via the petrosal sinuses represents an additional and important route leading to cavernous sinus thrombosis. If one keeps in mind that cerebral and meningeal veins also drain into the cavernous sinus, other serious complications such as brain abscess and spreading meningitis can be understood on the basis of retrograde spread. Signs of meningeal irritation such as rigidity of the neck and headache were present also in our case.

What anatomical features does the cavernous sinus share with other sinuses and in what respect does it differ? Like other intracranial venous sinuses it is located between two layers of dura, is lined by endothelium, but is lacking a muscular coat. It differs from other dural sinuses, however, in that it is traversed by numerous trabeculae, which give it a sponge-like appearance. This arrangement also makes it quite liable to thrombosis. Embedded in its lateral wall are the oculomotor, trochlear, and first and second divisions of the trigeminal nerve, while the internal carotid artery with its sympathetic plexus and the abducens nerve course through its lumen (Fig. 2).

Eye signs in cavernous sinus thrombosis

How do you explain the swelling of the eyelids and conjunctiva, the exophthalmos, the congestion of the retinal vessels,

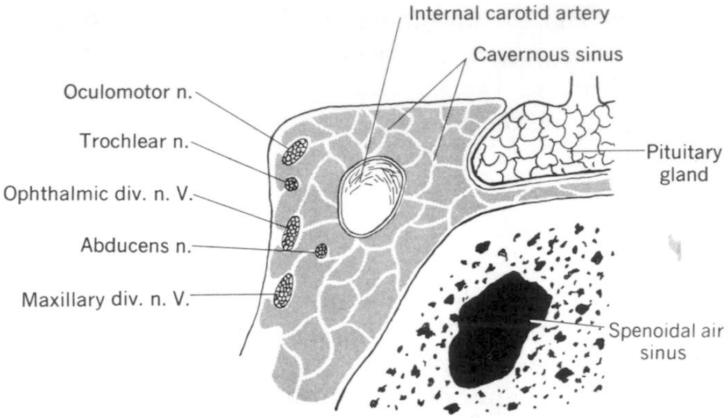

Figure 2 depicts a cross-section of the right cavernous sinus showing its important nerve and arterial contents.

and edema of the optic nerve in this patient? All these signs are caused by interference with the blood flow in the sinus and ophthalmic veins due to the thrombosis. The latter causes retrograde congestion of the ocular veins and edema (swelling) of the orbital structures. What signs do we have in our case that the right third, fourth, and sixth cranial nerves are affected by the sinus thrombosis? How would you test for specific involvement of the abducens and trochlear nerves? Detailed examination pertaining to function of individual eye muscles was difficult in our patient in view of the swelling of the right eye and his poor and irrational condition, but it was found that all voluntary movements of the eyeball were abolished. The oculomotor nerve supplies all muscles moving the eyeball with the exception of the superior oblique and lateral rectus muscles, which are innervated by the trochlear and abducens nerves, respectively. How would you test the functions of these two muscles? If the superior oblique is functionless due to involvement of the fourth cranial nerve, there is loss of downward movement of the eyeball if it is adducted. In case of paralysis of the lateral rectus there is loss of full abduction of the eyeball. Both of these motions were abolished in our case. The impairment of vision in the right eye can be explained on the basis of edema of the optic nerve, with congestion of the central vein of the retina which drains into the superior ophthalmic vein.

Are there clinical indications that the upper two divisions of the trigeminal nerve, which lie in the wall of the sinus, were also involved? There were sensory disturbances in the face along the distribution of these two divisions.

Later protrusion and swelling of the left eye with abducens paralysis indicate involvement of the left cavernous sinus also. Are there antomical pathways for the spread of the thrombosis from the right to the left sinus? The two cavernous sinuses are connected by anterior and posterior intercavernous sinuses which may readily spread the infection from one sinus to the other. The abducens nerve, being in a more exposed position within the sinus, is often the first of the nerves supplying the eye muscles to be involved in sinus thrombosis. Occasional reports of cases, that have come to autopsy, note infectious thrombosis of the internal carotid artery within the sinus. This of course could be the course of spread of infection to the brain by means of cerebral arterial branches.

The presence of positive blood cultures in our case indicates that the infection had spread beyond the confines of the cranium; the more gratifying is the final felicitous outcome of the case, which is not as common as one might expect in this era of vigorous antibiotic treatment. Disappearance of the local signs can be explained on the basis of subsidence of the infection and recanalization of the thrombosed sinus, as well as by development of a collateral circulation bypassing the sinus.

4 Cancer of the Lip with Lymphatic Spread

A 58-year-old farmer comes to the outpatient department with an ulcerated swelling involving parts of the red portion of the lower lip on the left. He states that the lesion started as a scab about six years earlier and that it gradually enlarged. From time to time it heals over, but then breaks open again and occasionally bleeds.

EXAMINATION

On examination the left portion of the lower lip shows an area of induration which is centrally ulcerated. The ulcer is about 2 cm. in its largest diameter, and is located at the vermilion border of the lower lip close to the left angle of the mouth. The borders of the ulcer are elevated and hard. When slightly scraped the ulcer bleeds readily. There are several hard, non-tender, enlarged nodes palpable in the left submandibular and carotid triangles. Otherwise examination is negative. Particularly is there no sign of involvement of other nodes besides the cervical nodes.

DIAGNOSIS

Cancer of the lip with probable metastasis to the cervical nodes. Biopsy of the primary lesion of the lip and needle biopsy of one of the enlarged submandibular nodes confirm the diagnosis of squamous cell cancer.

THERAPY

The patient is admitted to the hospital for surgery. Under general anesthesia using an endotracheal tube the primary ulcerated tumor is removed by a V-shaped excision, which includes a 5 mm.-wide margin of normal appearing tissue around the tumor. The defect is closed by a flap of approximately the same shape from the opposite surface of the upper lip, which is rotated around to form a new corner of the mouth.

The next step in the operation is a "radical neck dissection," which aims at removal of all deep cervical lymph nodes on the diseased side from the lower margin of the mandible to the clavicle, and from the midline and beyond it in the submental triangle to the anterior border of the trapezius. In depth it includes the lymphatics between the deep surface of the platysma and the prevertebral fascia.

The operation consists of removal in one block of the deep cervical lymphatics, particularly those in the submandibular and submental triangles, around the internal jugular vein and surrounding the accessory nerve and the transverse cervical vessels. The procedure includes sacrifice of the submandibular salivary gland, the sternocleidomastoid muscle, the accessory nerve, the internal jugular vein, the cutaneous branches of the cervical plexus, and the ansa cervicalis.

Skin flaps are widely reflected to expose the anterior and posterior triangles of the neck. The skin flaps include the platysma muscle. Attention is paid to preserving the marginal mandibular branch of the facial nerve where it courses along the lower margin of the mandible superficial to the facial artery and vein. These vessels are ligated and cut. The first structure encountered is the external jugular vein, which is ligated and resected to allow later removal of the sternocleidomastoid muscle, which this vein crosses superficially. The sternocleidomastoid muscle at the site of its distal attachment to sternum and clavicle and the posterior belly of the omohyoid are divided. The internal jugular vein is doubly ligated and severed just above the clavicle. Attention is paid to preservation of vagus and phrenic nerves and the trunks of the brachial plexus. The phrenic nerve and the trunks of the brachial plexus lie deep to the prevertebral fascia, which may or may not be removed in this operation. Likewise kept intact are the common, external, and internal carotid arteries and the thoracic duct on the left. The accessory nerve is cut close to its entrance into the trapezius muscle.

Next the surgeon removes all areolar and lymphatic tissue, starting in the posterior-inferior region of the posterior triangle and working his way forward and upward. Here the transverse cervical, and usually the suprascapular vessels are ligated and severed and the supraclavicular nerves cut. The other superficial sensory branches of the cervical plexus are also sacrificed at this time. As the bulk of tissues consisting of the sternocleidomastoid and omohyoid muscles, the internal jugular vein, and the areolar and fatty tissue with the lymphatics are reflected upward, the common carotid artery and its two divisions with the lower branches of the external carotid artery are exposed. The ansa cervicalis has been sacrificed previously to allow opening of the carotid sheath and removal of the internal jugular vein and adjacent lymph nodes. The important tributaries of the internal jugular vein are ligated and cut. The proximal end of the internal jugular vein is clamped, ligated, and sectioned as high as possible. Special care is taken again to avoid injury to the vagus nerve. The attachment of the sternocleidomastoid muscle to the mastoid process is cut as is the attachment of the omohyoid to the hyoid bone. The proximal end of the accessory nerve is likewise severed.

These steps are followed by removal of all fat and lymph nodes from the carotid, submental, and submandibular triangles. In the latter, the submandibular salivary gland is removed and its duct ligated, but care is taken not to injure the lingual and hypoglossal nerves. Removal of the submental nodes from the opposite side entails crossing the midline and requires exposure of the anterior belly of the opposite digastric muscle. The mass of tissue dissected out is removed in one block with the aim of eliminating all possibly cancerous lymphatics without cutting into them, thus avoiding dispersal of cancer cells.

After the dissection is completed, all bleeding is controlled by sutures and the wound is closed. A drain is left inside along the course of the common carotid artery and brought out through the surgical wound.

FURTHER COURSE

The postoperative course in this patient was uneventful. He was up and about the second day and was discharged from the hospital ten days later. Examination six months, one, two, and three years after surgery showed no signs of recurrence.

DISCUSSION

In the design of this operation it is realized that cancer of the lip spreads by way of the deep cervical lymphatics, but generally remains confined to the head and neck. Death from unchecked cancer occurs when large masses of cancerous cervical nodes interfere with swallowing, thus leading to gradual starvation, or slowly compress the air passages, thus strangling the patient, or when these cancerous nodes erode the great vessels resulting in an acute and profuse fatal hemorrhage. Hence, the goal of the radical neck dissection is removal of all deep cervical lymph nodes which may harbor metastatic cancer cells having arrived there by way of lymphatic vessels.

Lymphatic drainage of lower lip

What is the lymphatic drainage of the lower lip? The lymph vessels from the lateral portion of the lip pass downward to submandibular nodes of the same side in the submandibular triangle, while the more medial portions of the lip drain in part also to submental nodes in the submental triangle to both sides of the midline. While lymph vessels, even from the lateral portions of the lower lip, may cross the midline to submental nodes of the other side, the danger of contralateral spread is greater the closer the lesion is to the midline (Fig. 1). The possibility of this spread is the rationale for removing all

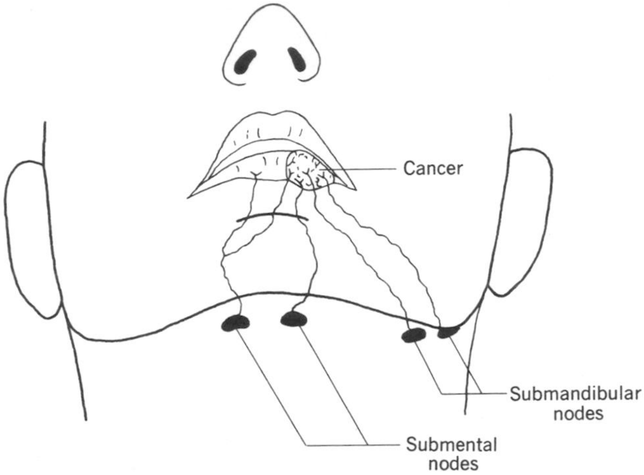

Figure 1 shows cancer of the lower lip with first relay of potentially involved lymph nodes.

lymph nodes in the submental triangle to both sides of the midline as was done in our case. The submandibular and submental nodes represent the first relay station of the lymphatics of the lower lip.

Name the further lymphatic channels along which cancer of the lower lip would spread after it invaded the submandibular and/or submental nodes, or with which an occasional lymph vessel from the lip, that bypasses these nodes, would connect. The chain of deep cervical nodes is the final pathway into which all lymph vessels from head and neck drain. It consists of a large and variable number of lymph nodes that are related to the carotid sheath and particularly to the internal jugular vein. Many of these lie directly under the sternocleidomastoid muscle (Fig. 2). This is the reason that this important vein and the sternocleidomastoid muscle have to be resected in order not to leave any potentially cancerous lymph structures behind that are in close contact with them. The omohyoid muscle, which is likewise sacrificed, divides this chain into a superior and inferior group at the site where it crosses the

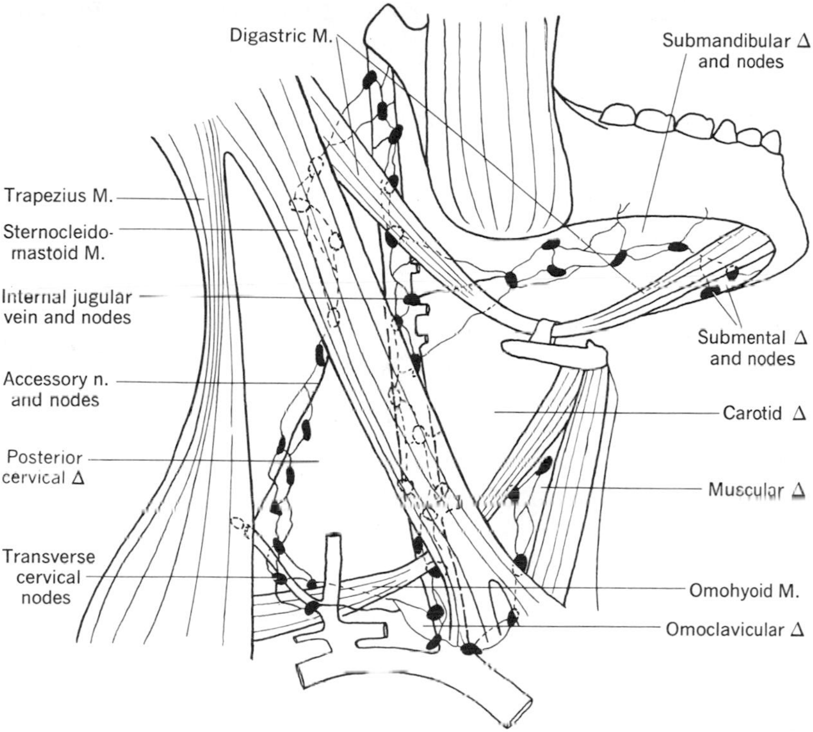

Figure 2 shows cervical triangles and deep cervical lymph nodes.

internal jugular vein. Occasionally, and if the surgeon is reasonably certain that cancerous invasion has not progressed beyond the superior deep cervical lymph nodes, a supraomohyoid dissection is done which carries the dissection only to the crossing point of the omohyoid muscle. The superior deep cervical nodes drain in part into the inferior nodes, part of their efferent vessels contribute to the formation of the jugular trunk which receives the lymph from the inferior deep cervical group. A number of deep cervical nodes occupy a position away from the internal jugular chain around the accessory nerve and the transverse cervical and suprascapular vessels (Fig. 2). The removal of these nodes therefore entails sacrifice of this important motor nerve and these vessels.

Triangles of the neck and their lymph nodes

In the radical neck dissection what six triangles of the neck are encompassed from which all fatty areolar and lymphatic tissue is removed? All triangles of the neck are involved in this operation: the submandibular, the submental, the carotid, and the muscular triangles, which are all parts of the anterior triangle, and the posterior cervical and omoclavicular (subclavian) subdivisions of the posterior triangle. Identify the boundaries of these triangles from Figure 2. Are lymph nodes present in all these triangles and where are they most prevalent? The submental and submandibular nodes are present in the triangles of the same name. The nodes in the unpaired submental triangle lie on the mylohyoid muscle between the anterior bellies of the digastric muscles. Why does the submandibular salivary gland and its duct have to be sacrificed in the removal of the submandibular lymph nodes? These nodes lie within the fascial sheath of and in close relation to this salivary gland and cannot be removed properly without removal of the gland. The close relationship of some of the smaller lymph nodes in this group to the facial vessels necessitates ligation and sacrifice of these vessels. Most of the superior deep cervical nodes lie in the carotid triangle and deep to the sternocleidomastoid muscle. A number of nodes of the cervical chain overflow into the muscular triangle and the two divisions of the posterior triangle. In the latter are located the important nodes around the accessory nerve and the transverse cervical and suprascapular vessels (Fig. 2). Again this entails removal of this nerve and ligation and sacrifice of these vessels. Of what vessels are the transverse cervical and suprascapular arteries and veins branches and tributaries? The arteries are branches of the thyrocervical trunk of the subclavian artery, and the veins are tributaries of the external jugular vein, which is likewise ligated and removed. How does this latter vein drain? It is the only tributary of the subclavian vein.

Loss of internal jugular vein

The most important structure that has to be sacrified is the internal jugular vein including its tributaries, particularly the lingual, the pharyngeal, the facial, the superior and middle thyroid, and the occipital veins. If one realizes that the internal jugular vein is the largest vein of the head and neck draining blood from the brain, the face, and neck and that the external jugular vein, which also drains part of the head and neck, is likewise removed, one is surprised that the loss of these veins is generally well tolerated. One might ask why total extirpation of the internal jugular vein from the site of its cranial exit to the level of the clavicle is necessary. All surgeons who have participated in the design of radical neck dissection, agree upon the need for removal of this vein. It is surrounded by cervical lymph nodes which may readily be adherent to it and which cannot be completely eliminated without concomitant resection of the vein.

How is venous drainage from the head and neck effectuated after ligation of the internal jugular vein? Due to ample communications across the midline, the contralateral internal jugular vein will easily adjust to the additional blood flow into it. The vertebral venous plexus also participates in the venous drainage from the brain and other parts of the head. There may be a transient, harmless increase in intracranial pressure after unilateral ligation of the internal jugular vein, but only in rare cases will there be a serious rise reflected in headache, slow pulse, and high blood pressure. Lumbar puncture is the treatment of choice in these cases.

Motor and sensory nerves sacrificed in radical neck dissection

What muscles does the accessory nerve supply? The accessory nerve supplies two important muscles in the field of this operation, the sternocleidomastoid and the trapezius muscle, of which the former is resected during the operation. How does denervation of the trapezius affect the patient? Generally, loss of function of the trapezius is well tolerated although noticeable by a slight shoulder drop. It is possible that some motor function remains in this muscle since it may receive additional motor fibers from the third and fourth cervical nerves which otherwise furnish proprioceptive fibers to the trapezius muscle. What muscles could replace the action of the trapezius in elevating and retracting the scapula? The levator scapulae and the rhomboid muscles are synergists of the trapezius in this action. What other motor nerves are resected in this operation and what muscles do they supply? The ansa cervicalis (hypoglossi) lying on or in the anterior layer of the carotid sheath has to be sacrificed. It supplies the infrahyoid muscles, whose denervation on one side is well tolerated. Attention is paid to preservation of one small motor nerve—the marginal mandibular branch of the facial nerve, which runs along the lower edge of the mandible just superficial to the site of crossing of the bone by the facial vessels which are ligated. If it has to be resected, it results in some disfigurement in the region of the mouth, particularly when smiling.

What sensory nerves are sacrificed? Where are they located and of what are they branches? The cutaneous branches of the cervical plexus are removed in the dissection of the posterior triangle, where they are placed quite superficially. They are the lesser occipital, the greater auricular, the transverse cervical, and the supraclavicular nerves, all derived from ventral rami of C2 to C4. The resulting anesthesia and numbness is well tolerated and gradually decreases. How do you explain this? It can be assumed that sensory nerves in the neighborhood gradually take over the function in the desensitized area by sending fibers into it. What nerves would be most likely to participate in this sensory supply? It would be particularly the cutaneous branches of the dorsal rami of cervical nerves II to IV. It is also conceivable that nerve fibers from the distal end of the central stump may gradually grow out and reach the skin to reassume its sensory innervation.

Attention should of course be paid to the preservation of the vagus. What is its relation to the internal jugular vein and the common and internal carotid arteries? It lies medial to the vein and lateral to the arteries and on a somewhat deeper plane. Would section of the vagus nerve on one side be fatal? Injury of one vagus nerve is not followed by serious cardiac or pulmonary complications but will result in unilateral vocal cord paralysis with partial obstruction of the air passages. This complication will require watchful nursing care with particular attention to the air passages and tracheostomy in case of breathing difficulties.

In the rather difficult dissection of the submandibular triangle, attention is paid to avoidance of injury to the hypoglossal and lingual nerves. Removal of the submandibular salivary gland and duct, of all areolar tissue and lymph nodes, as well as ligation of the facial vessels facilitate display of these important nerves. Quite frequently the lower pole of the parotid gland is also amputated, and some surgeons recommend the separation of the posterior belly of the digastric and stylohyoid muscles from the hyoid bone and their resection. What muscles form the floor of the submandibular triangle which have to be defined in this operation? Portions of the mylohyoid and the hyoglossus muscles are the deep boundary of the triangle, with the mylohyoid overlapping the hyoglossus superficially. In the area where the two muscles overlap, do the lingual and hypoglossal nerves run superficial to the mylohyoid, deep to it, that is, between it and the hyoglossus muscle, or deep to the hyoglossus? They run between mylohyoid and hyoglossus muscles, with the lingual nerve cranial to the hypoglossal nerve and with the duct of the submandibular gland between them. The hypoglossal nerve before its disappearance between the two muscles is exposed to injury while it makes a loop into the carotid triangle caudal to the posterior belly of the digastric muscle, before it returns to the submandibular triangle crossing deep to the digastric muscle.

5 Tracheostomy

An 11-month-old infant girl is brought to the emergency room of the hospital with a history of cough of two days' duration and noisy respiratory efforts. The infant seems to struggle for air and appears very frightened.

EXAMINATION

On examination, the face and particularly the lips display bluish discoloration (cyanosis), the nostrils dilate with every breath, and the child struggles for air. In breathing, the accessory muscles of respiration are also utilized. The infant has a rapid pulse and a temperature of 101°. From time to time she has noisy coughing spells. The throat and larynx appear red and inflamed. On auscultation of the chest, coarse rales (abnormal respiratory sounds) are heard over the chest.

DIAGNOSIS

Acute inflammation of the upper respiratory passages, including trachea and bronchi, with swelling of the mucosa, resulting in partial obstruction of the air passages.

THERAPY

The infant is placed in a steam tent to create a highly humid environment, and expectoration is induced by medication to

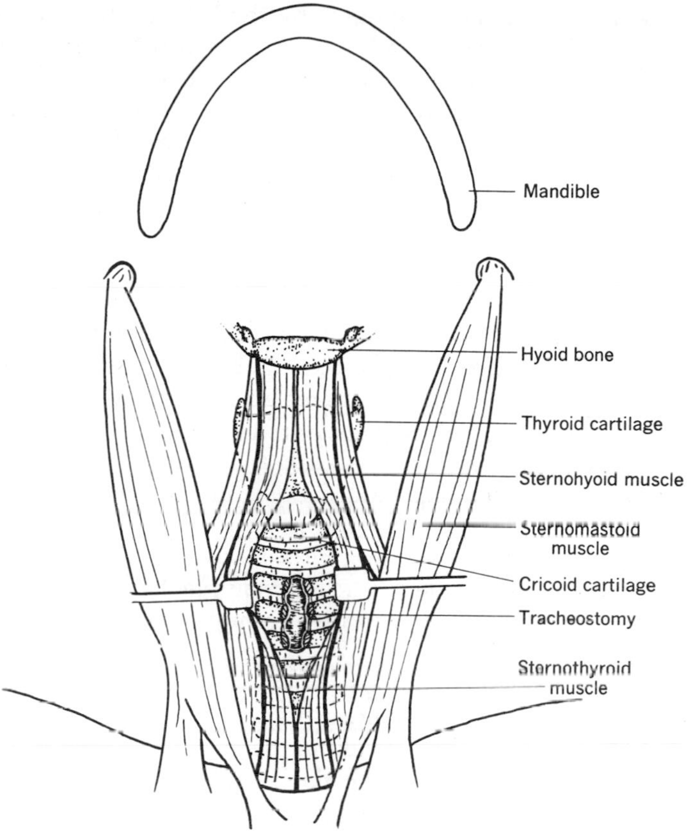

Figure 1 shows site of tracheostomy in second, third, and fourth tracheal cartilages. Notice structures in the midline above tracheostomy site. Infrahyoid muscles are retracted.

expel the mucus blocking the air passages. Later, oxygen and antibiotics are administered. In spite of these procedures, the infant becomes more restless and the cyanotic discoloration increases. The face has a very anxious expression and she seems to become more exhausted and weaker. The infant is therefore sent to the operating room and prepared for tracheostomy.

Local anesthesia is applied to the site of the projected incision. The patient's head is overextended by placing a sandbag under her shoulders. A nurse is stationed at the head of the table to see that rotation of the infant's head is avoided. A transverse incision is made one fingerbreadth above the jugular (suprasternal) notch and is about 3 cm. in length. This incision passes through the skin, superficial fascia, platysma, and the superficial (investing) layer of the cervical fascia. These structures are widely retracted to give ample access to the area. All superficial veins encountered in the field are ligated and divided. The fascia over the infrahyoid muscles is incised from the thyroid cartilage to the jugular notch of the sternum, and the infrahyoid muscles are retracted laterally. The isthmus of the thyroid gland is pulled cranialward. The pretracheal fascia is incised and the second, third, and fourth tracheal cartilages are identified and divided in the midline together with the mucosal lining of the trachea (Fig. 1). The margins of the tracheal incision are spread apart by hooks and the opening in the trachea (tracheostomy) enlarged. A mucous plug is expelled spontaneously through the opening in the trachea. The infant takes a deep breath followed by a deep sigh. A tracheostomy tube is then inserted. The upper and lower ends of the subcutaneous incision are closed by sutures. The tracheostomy tube is held in place by a loose tape around the neck. The margins of the skin wound and the area around the tube are covered with moist gauze dressings.

FURTHER COURSE

The infant is placed in an oxygen tent, and the air is humidified to keep the mucous membrane of the trachea moist and to prevent secretions from drying out. The inner tube of the tracheostomy tube is removed and cleaned frequently, and suction of the trachea is employed to aspirate mucus. Antibiotics are given. Within the next ten days the respiratory infection subsides. Prior to removal of the tracheostomy tube, the lumen of the tube is obstructed in gradual stages by being plugged over two- to three-day periods, using first a cork obstructing only 50 per cent of the lumen and then a full plug. The child is discharged as cured.

DISCUSSION

We are dealing here with an infant in severe respiratory distress. How do you explain the blue discoloration (cyanosis) which is particularly noticeable on the lips? The cyanosis is due to insufficient oxygenation of blood in the lungs and can be most easily detected by inspection of the lips where a translucent epithelium covers a rich network of blood vessels.

What are the accessory muscles of respiration which are utilized in case of respiratory difficulties? In dyspnea (shortness of breath) the auxiliary muscles of respiration are called into action to add their strength to the normal muscular and mechanical elements which effect breathing by alternating changes in the craniocaudal, transverse, and anteroposterior diameters of the chest. In forced inspiration the scaleni, the sternocleidomastoid, the serratus anterior, and the pectoralis major and pectoralis minor muscles increase the capacity of the thorax, the latter three acting on the ribs, with the shoulder girdle and arms being fixed by the action of other muscles. The inspiratory widening of the nasal opening in our case is an indication that all available muscles are called upon to assist in breathing.

In forced expiration maximal contraction of the abdominal muscles is called into play to enhance the action of the normal expulsive forces.

Tracheostomy, or tracheotomy, as it was called in the past, is the surgical formation of an artificial opening in the trachea. Tracheostomy is indicated in our case in order to establish an open airway in the presence of inflammatory laryngeal obstruction and to evacuate tracheobronchial secretions which block the windpipe further down.

What is the purpose of overextension of the neck at the time of surgery? Will the normal curve of the cervical part of the spinal column be enhanced or decreased by this maneuver? Why is close attention paid to avoidance of rotation of head and neck?

The advantage of overextension is a lengthening of the trachea, which is pulled out of the mediastinum, a forward displacement of the trachea into the operative field by the increased anterior convexity of the cervical portion of the spinal column, and a tensening of the skin and fascia, which facilitates a clean-cut incision. Straightening of the neck will line up the superior notch of the thyroid cartilage, the trachea, and the jugular notch of the sternum in a straight line for better identification of the trachea. On the other hand, rotation of head and neck, particularly under emergency conditions, leads to displacement of the trachea, and may possibly induce the operator to miss the trachea entirely and insert the tracheostomy tube into the lax paratracheal connective tissue.

Cervical fascia encountered in tracheostomy

In addition to the superficial fascia which may contain fair amounts of subcutaneous fat, what fascial layers are encountered in this operation?

With the exception of the superficial fascia, all fascial layers present in the anterior triangle of the neck are derivatives of the deep fascia of the neck, the cervical fascia. The first fascial layer that is incised in approaching the trachea, after skin and superficial fascia have been retracted, is the superficial (investing) layer of the cervical fascia. This layer bridges the anterior triangle as a sheet with offshoots that surround the infrahyoid muscles. The superficial layer of the cervical fascia splits caudally to attach to both anterior and posterior aspects of the manubrium of the sternum, thus forming a space that extends upward for a variable distance. It is therefore frequently opened in tracheostomy. What are the contents of this suprasternal space? In addition to fat and some lymph nodes, it contains an important anastomosis between the right and left anterior jugular veins, often called the jugular arch.

Identify the two pairs of infrahyoid muscles which are closest to the midline in the area of the operation and which have to be retracted. Which one of these muscle pairs almost reaches the midline just about the jugular notch of the sternum? The sternohyoid is the more superficial, and the sternothyroid is the deeper, but it is the sternothyroid muscles that converge from the thyroid cartilage to the midline at the site of their attachment to the posterior surface of the manubrium sterni, and thus narrow the operative field, if a low tracheostomy is undertaken (Fig. 1).

The next fascial layer which has to be divided is the pretracheal fascia, another derivative of the cervical fascia. It covers the larynx and trachea, and forms a sheath for the thyroid gland. It continues caudally behind the sternum into the mediastinum.

Landmarks in the midline

With the cutting of the pretracheal fascia the level of the respiratory tube has been reached, and it is now indicated to review the important landmarks in the infrahyoid part of the midline of the neck. Identify these on yourself by palpation and with the help of a mirror and point them out, passing from cranially to caudally.

The hyoid bone is a subcutaneous structure and can easily be felt and moved from side to side. Caudal to the hyoid bone, and connected to it by the thyrohyoid membrane, is the thyroid cartilage, characterized by the laryngeal prominence in the midline, the "Adam's apple," with the laminae of the thyroid on each side of this prominence. They form the superior thyroid notch just cranial to the prominence. Caudal to the thyroid cartilage we palpate the arch of the cricoid cartilage. Connecting these two cartilages in the middle is the strong cricothyroid ligament. Below the cricoid cartilage are the tracheal rings which give the trachea its corrugated surface. Partly masking the trachea in the midline is the isthmus of the thyroid, which overlaps the second and third, and sometimes the fourth tracheal rings. The trachea recedes as it descends toward the mediastinum, and in the adult lies 4 cm. from the surface at the cranial border of the manubrium.

In infants the neck is, of course, very short so that the field of operation is quite small. The isthmus of the thyroid gland can easily be dislodged by retracting it upward or downward and snipping through the loose fibrous tissue that attaches it to the trachea. It can also be bisected and the parts retracted after ligation of bleeding vessels.

Larynx, trachea, and esophagus

If the site of tracheostomy is not properly identified by palpation, tracheostomy may be done too far cranially. In that case, the cricoid and even the thyroid cartilages may be damaged, and laryngeal stenosis and severe interference with the voice may result.

Are the cartilaginous rings of the trachea complete, or are they deficient in some portion of their circumference? The approximately twenty rings of hyaline cartilage, which form the supporting framework of the trachea, occupy only two-thirds of the tracheal circumference, being U-shaped and open posteriorly. The so-called membranous portion of the trachea, consisting of fibrous connective tissues and smooth muscles, closes this gap.

Does the absence of firm cartilage from the posterior wall of the trachea have any bearing on complications of tracheostomy? What organ lies in immediate apposition to the posterior aspect of the trachea, only a small amount of areolar tissue intervening? The posterior membranous portion of the trachea may be perforated, particularly in emergency operations, and a tracheo-esophageal communication may be established. This accident is frequently fatal, since milk and solid food may be aspirated into the lung through this fistula. This complication is more apt to occur in infants because of the small size of the trachea, whose diameter may be still further reduced by the protrusion of the anterior esophageal wall into the lumen of the trachea during swallowing and coughing spells. In small children, under emergency conditions, even the anterior surface of the vertebral column has been injured by the knife of the surgeon.

Recently a suggestion has been made by military medical circles, concerned with disaster care, to have paramedical personnel trained in establishing an artificial airway through the cricothyroid membrane as a lifesaving operation under adverse and catastrophic conditions. If this pathway is utilized, is there the same danger of posterior perforation with regard to the cricoid cartilage? The cricoid cartilage, which is located immediately above the beginning of the trachea, is a closed ring, which has a large cartilaginous plate posteriorly protecting the air passage at this level against posterior perforation. The value of this method is still open to question.

Complications of tracheostomy

One of the most troublesome and occasionally fatal complications of tracheostomy, particularly when done under emergency conditions, is hemorrhage from veins and arteries. Since it is one of the prime requirements of an orderly tracheostomy to stay in the midline, the first question that arises is: Are there blood vessels of any size in the midline that may be endangered? The following structures are noteworthy (Fig. 2): (1) The communication between the anterior jugular veins, that cross the midline within the suprasternal space, has been mentioned previously. (2) The left brachiocephalic vein is apt to be located above the jugular notch in infants and children and may cause technical difficulties and severe complications in low tracheostomy. (3) The inferior thyroid vein, instead of being paired, may be unpaired, or the right and left veins may unite to form a single large vein that runs in the midline and generally drains into the left brachiocephalic vein. (4) In 10 per cent of all subjects there arises an additional artery to the thyroid gland from either the brachiocephalic trunk, the arch of the aorta, or the right common carotid artery. It is named the lowest thyroid, or thyroid ima artery, and can be quite large. It may ascend in the midline in front of the trachea on its way to the thyroid gland, and may complicate

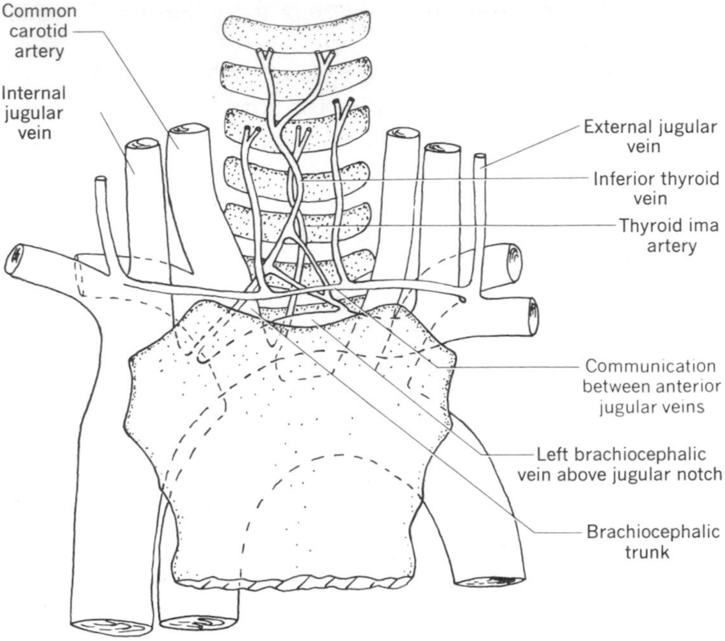

Figure 2 shows potential sites of blood vessel injuries in tracheostomy as listed in text.

the operation. (5) Very occasionally the brachiocephalic trunk (innominate artery) may ascend above the jugular notch and be endangered in the operation. (6) It is hard to conceive, and only understandable if emergency conditions in a very restless, suffocating child are visualized, that the common carotid artery or internal jugular vein may be lacerated. But such cases have been reported.

What large muscle protects these vessels in front and prevents their injury in tracheostomy, if this muscle with all its underlying structures is retracted out of the way? The sternocleidomastoid muscle overlies and protects the carotid sheath and its contents. It should, of course, be realized that, under proper operating room conditions, venous hemorrhage and bleeding from an injured thyroid ima artery can be controlled by ligation of the damaged vessel without any further consequences to the patient.

In infants a large thymus may protrude into the neck in front of the trachea and cause some operative difficulties in low tracheostomy.

If the skin is too tightly closed around the tracheostomy tube, expired air may be forced into the tissues of the neck, causing a subcutaneous accumulation of air (emphysema) in the loose tissue of the cervical region. Is it anatomically possible for this air to leak gradually downward into the mediastinum and cause circulatory embarrassment by compressing the large vessels of the mediastinum? The loose connective tissue of the neck is continued into the mediastinum in so-called fascial spaces, which are spaces bounded by the various layers of the cervical fascia, so that penetration of the air into the mediastinum is a frequent complication of cervical emphysema. If mediastinal emphysema is disregarded and remains untreated, the air may rupture into the pleural cavity and cause air filling of the pleural sac (pneumothorax). If this happens on both sides, it may quickly become fatal. A one-sided pneumothorax can also be produced by inadvertent injury to the dome of the pleura in an emergency tracheostomy. Infection may likewise travel from the site of the tracheostomy down into the mediastinum and cause serious complications.

6 Torticollis

A five-year-old girl is brought to the pediatrician by her mother with the complaint that since early childhood the right side of her neck has been twisted and deformed. On inquiry, the mother states that childbirth was prolonged and difficult and that delivery took place with buttocks presenting first (breech delivery). Within a few weeks after birth, the mother noticed a spindle-shaped swelling over the right side of the infant's neck which was very tender on touch and on passive movement of the head. During the next few months the swelling and tenderness over the area gradually subsided. Later on, when the child was about one year old, the large muscle at the right side of the neck appeared cord-like. Gradually and progressively the neck became stiff and deformed with the head tilted toward the right side and the face turned toward the left. The face also became asymmetrical (Fig. 1).

EXAMINATION

On examination the child appears somewhat underdeveloped and poorly nourished. On request the child is unable to straighten her head, even with the assistance of the examiner. In moving the head the right sternocleidomastoid muscle appears contracted and transformed into a fibrous cord. The head is drawn toward the right shoulder; the chin is elevated and

The term torticollis means "twisted neck."

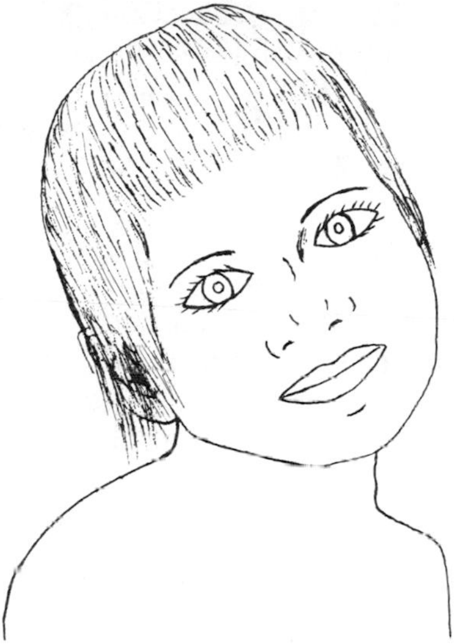

Figure 1—Shows right-sided torticollis in a young girl. Notice that the head is drawn toward the right shoulder, the elevated chin points to the left.

points toward the left. The facial asymmetry consists of shortening of the skull and face on the right side in an anteroposterior direction, a flattening of the lateral aspect of the face, and an uneven level of the eyes. Further examination and roentgenograms reveal that the patient has a left-convex scoliosis in the lower cervical and upper thoracic region, and a compensatory right-convex scoliosis in the middle and lower thoracic area.

DIAGNOSIS

Congenital wry-neck or torticollis.

THERAPY

In view of the long duration of the condition, surgery is decided upon. Under general anesthesia, the platysma and anterior layer of the general investing (enveloping) fascia over the sternocleidomastoid muscle are divided. The muscle is seen to be transformed into a dense, fibrous band. The fibrotic muscle with its two heads is then excised, attention being paid to avoidance of injury to the underlying accessory nerve and the major vessels deep to the muscle. The head is gradually manipulated into the correct position. The posterior layer of the enveloping fascia, which covers the posterior aspect of the muscle, also appears taut and shortened. Portions of this posterior layer are also excised. The wound is closed. The head is kept in a splinting harness for several weeks. Active and passive stretching exercises are then carried out. The child is seen six months later with the head being in the normal position. There is no obvious evidence of loss of motion of head and neck.

DISCUSSION

Obviously we are dealing here with a congenital condition that has transformed the sternocleidomastoid muscle into a nonfunctioning cord. By its rigidity and shortening, this cord has distorted the position of the head and neck and has brought about alterations in growth of the face. In order to understand this not uncommon entity of congenital torticollis, we have to realize that it is primarily confined to the sternocleidomastoid muscle. All other deformities are secondary in character and result from the abnormal position of the head.

Normal function of the sternocleidomastoid muscle

What is the normal function of the sternocleidomastoid muscle, or to use a shorter term, the "sternomastoid" muscle? Its function is rather complex but can be deducted from its origin and insertion. The origin of the muscle is by two heads from the front of the manubrium sterni and the medial third of the clavicle. The sternal head is tendinous, the clavicular head more fleshy and tendinous only at its immediate site of origin. The lateral head passes deep to the medial, but the two combine about the middle of the neck and the fibers from the two origins cannot be separated as the muscle approaches its insertion. The muscle takes a spiral turn around the lateral side of the neck to its insertion into the mastoid process and into the lateral half of the superior nuchal line of the occiput. Notice that the muscle at its origin faces forward, at its insertion, laterally. Consequently, the course of the muscle from its origin to its insertion is directed obliquely upward, posteriorly and laterally. The effect of the shortening and scarring of the muscle on the position of the head in our case accurately simulates one-sided contraction of the normal muscle. The muscle inclines the head to its own side and rotates it in such a way that the chin points upward and to the opposite side (Figs. 1 and 2). If the purpose of one-sided movement is simple rotation of the head in the atlanto-axial joint around a vertical axis through the dens of the axis, without lateral bending of the head towards the shoulder, part of the effect of sternomastoid contraction can be suppressed by activation of the opposite lateral flexors of the cervical spinal column such as the longus capitis, semispinalis capitis and cervicis, and splenius capitis, as well as scalenus medius.

Coming now to the combined action of both sternomastoids, it has to be realized that the main portion of the insertion of the muscles is posterior to the transverse axis, passing through the two atlanto-occipital joints, and that contraction of the two muscles will therefore result in extension of the head, i.e. a posterior tilt (Fig. 2). Other results of contraction of both muscles depend partly on the position of the head at the time of contraction and on combination with simultaneous contraction of other muscles. If, for example, the subject is lifting himself from the supine position as in rising from his bed, the more anterior fibers of the muscle in front of the transverse axis through the atlanto-occipital joint will assist the flexors of the cervical spinal column in flexing the head (Fig. 2). Bed-fast patients in a weakened condition are often unable to do so and need to be supported. In emaciated patients, the contracted sternomastoid muscles often stand out, as they try to lift themselves from their bed.

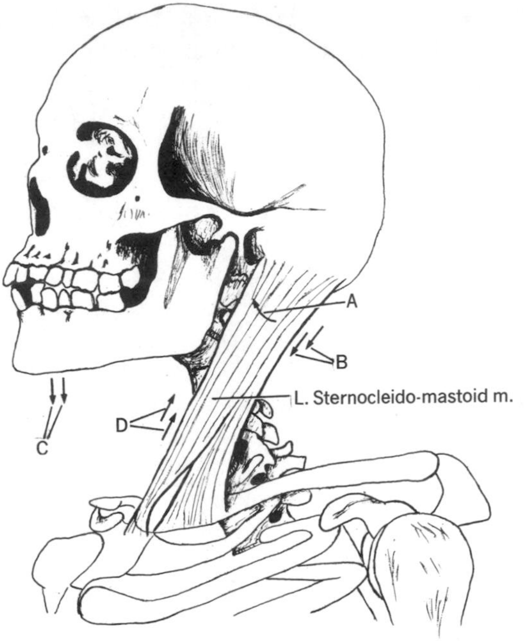

Figure 2—Action of sternocleidomastoid muscle. (Single arrow denotes one-sided contraction, double arrows indicate contraction of right and left muscles.) "A" refers to motion of left muscle in rotating head to right side with chin pointing upward. In one-sided contraction the head also is bent to side of muscle. "B" indicates extension of head when both muscles are contracted. "C" indicates flexion of head by sternocleidomastoid muscles in co-operation with flexors of the cervical spinal column. "D" shows muscles acting as accessory muscles of inspiration by raising manubrium of sternum when head is fixed by other muscles.

Finally, the muscle has to be regarded as an auxiliary muscle of inspiration if it acts from its insertion to the mastoid and superior nuchal line on its origin with the head being fixed by other muscles (Fig. 2).

In trying to understand the action of an individual muscle, such as the sternomastoid, it must be realized that in the living no muscle ever contracts by itself, that on the contrary, all movements such as flexion and extension, rotation and lateral bending of the head, require the co-operation of groups of other muscles, and that loss of function of one muscle is generally compensated for by the action of other muscles. This explains why our patient tolerated the excision of the muscle well. Similarly, the resection of the pectoralis major and minor muscles in radical surgery for cancer of the breast leads to surprisingly minor deficiencies of motion.

Nerve-supply of sternomastoid muscle

The nerve supply to the sternocleidomastoid muscle originates essentially from the accessory nerve (xi), and in part also from the ventral rami of cervical II and III. The latter nerves, however, may be purely proprioceptive in function.

Why does the accessory nerve have to be protected in surgery for torticollis if the muscle supplied by it is being excised anyhow? The accessory nerve also supplies all or the major portion of the trapezius, which of course is preserved in this operation.

Causes of congenital torticollis

As to the various and frequently disputed theories pertaining to the cause of congenital torticollis, many interesting applications of anatomy enter into this discussion.

Arterial supply of the muscle: A number of authors have ascribed the condition to arterial occlusion or partial interference with the arterial supply of the muscle during delivery, resulting in secondary scarring of the insufficiently nourished muscle. Actually numerous arterial branches ramify in the muscle and the blood supply is rather profuse. While the arteries supplying the muscle show variations in their number and course, the following named arteries have been given as a source of blood supply to the muscle: the posterior auricular, occipital, and superior thyroid arteries from the external carotid, in addition to a frequently mentioned direct muscular branch from the external carotid, and the transverse cervical and suprascapular arteries from the thyrocervical trunk of the subclavian artery.

These arteries form a plexus within the substance of the muscle in such a way that the branches originating from the external carotid supply the superior and middle portions, while the vessels coming from the thyrocervical trunk carry blood to the lower part of the muscle. All these branches, however, communicate with each other, along ascending and descending branches throughout the muscle belly. With the original sources of the arterial supply being so widely separated, it is hardly conceivable that interference with one artery or a limited number of arteries during delivery can result in such widespread and diffuse degeneration. One author also noted that in surgical removal of the diseased muscle, all arterial branches bled freely within the substance of the muscle.

Venous drainage of the muscle: A second cause given for congenital torticollis is venous occlusion during labor with resulting necrosis (cell death). Actually, the veins draining the muscle are even more numerous than the arteries supplying it. These veins are tributaries of all major neck veins. They consist of veins accompanying the arteries mentioned previously, and direct tributaries to the external, internal, and anterior jugular veins. There are broad communications between these veins, not only on the surface of the muscle, but also by means of a well-developed intramuscular plexus so that the areas drained by these veins widely overlap.

Most plausible cause of congenital torticollis: Other hypotheses pertaining to the cause of congenital torticollis have been offered but are unconvincing. It is interesting that 50 per cent of all cases of this disorder are breech deliveries. In the light of this and convincing histologic changes in the muscle at the time of operation in early infancy before maximal scarring of the muscle takes place, the most plausible explanation seems to be the following: the torticollis dates back to intrauterine malposition of the fetal head which in a few cases has also been demonstrated *in utero* by roentgenograms. This malposition subjects the muscle to undue pressure against the shoulder at a time when the muscle undergoes active growth and differentiation. The malposition also prevents normal entrance of the fetal head into the pelvis, resulting in breech presentation and other abnormal and prolonged types of delivery. Further trauma to the already deformed muscle at the time of birth ensues.

The later swelling of the muscle, observed in our and other cases, is the result of an inflammatory reaction to the prolonged birth trauma. However, cases have been reported in the literature where torticollis was present in babies that were delivered by Caeserian section and thus not exposed to birth trauma.

7 Whiplash Injury of Neck

A 52-year-old female schoolteacher comes to her physician's office, complaining of headaches, neck pain, and stiffness in the neck. These symptoms started four months ago after an automobile accident. Her car stopped at a street crossing and was struck from behind by another car. She states that at the time of the accident she was badly shaken up and developed immediate pain in the neck which radiated into both shoulders and gradually increased in intensity during the next few days. Since then, the shoulder pain has slowly diminished in intensity, but the other symptoms still persist.

EXAMINATION

On examination, the head is held rather rigid, apparently due to muscle spasm. Flexion, extension, and lateral rotation of head and neck cause pain and are resisted by the patient. There is some local tenderness on palpation, particularly over the area of the fourth and fifth cervical vertebra. Thorough X-ray examination shows disappearance of the normal cervical lordosis. There are slight degenerative changes at the lower cervical vertebrae with some bony spurs, particularly around the intervertebral foramina between C4 and C5; but the radiologist states that these alterations could be in keeping with the age of the patient. The most important roentgenographic finding is the absence of any signs of fracture of the cervical vertebrae.

DIAGNOSIS

Cervical syndrome due to hyperextension—hyperflexion (whiplash) injury caused by rear-end collision.

FURTHER COURSE AND THERAPY

The patient is given a sponge rubber neck collar which she is told to wear intermittently. Hot moist packs are applied by the patient herself at home, while dry heat is given in the office by means of short-wave therapy. Treatment also includes intermittent traction. Muscle relaxants and sedation are prescribed. Under this treatment the symptoms of the patient gradually improve, though some intermittent pain still remains but appears tolerable.

DISCUSSION

The term "whiplash" injury refers to the mechanism of the trauma, not to the underlying lesion, and is used to indicate the rapid change in motion from hyperextension of the head and the upper part of the neck to hyperflexion in rear-end collisions, and from extreme flexion to maximal extension in head-on collisions. The analogy to a whip refers to the more flexible upper part of the cervical spine acting as the lash, and the more fixed lower portion as the handle of the whip. Lately the term has fallen into disrepute, not only because the analogy of the cervical spine and superimposed heavy head to a whip is rather vague (if not mechanically incorrect), but also because it does not give any clue to the quite variable underlying pathology.

The tissue damage may range from a muscle strain or sprain of the cervical ligaments, to rupture of the ligaments and of the intervertebral disks, fractures of the vertebrae, pressure on and injury to the cervical cord and emerging cervical nerves, and damage to the vertebral artery with resulting interference with cerebral circulation.

The term "cervical syndrome due to rear-end or head-on collision" is now preferred by most authors. The broad spec-

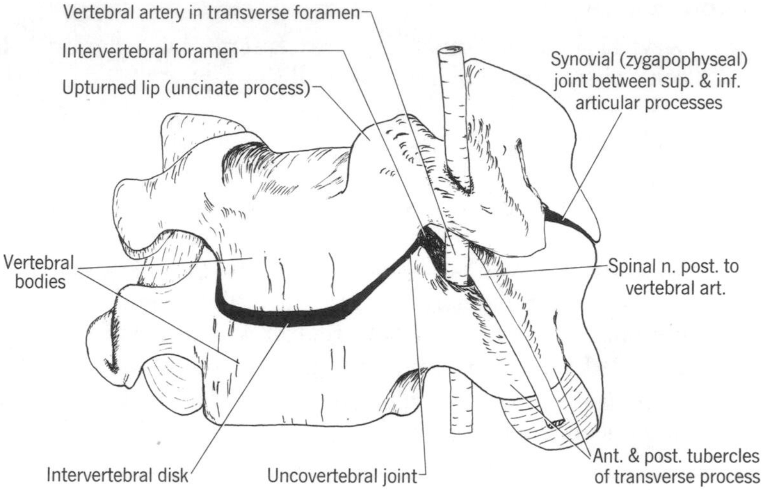

Figure 1—Oblique view of two articulated cervical vertebrae showing, anterior to the intervertebral foramen, the cartilaginous joint between vertebral bodies with the intervertebral disk and also the uncovertebral joint, and posterior to the intervertebral foramen the synovial joint between articular processes. Notice vertebral artery passing through the transverse foramen in front of the cervical nerve which emerges from the intervertebral foramen.

trum of injuries to the various tissues with possible involvement of muscles, ligaments, cartilage, bone, spinal cord, peripheral nerve structures, and blood vessels requires familiarity with the underlying anatomy.

Underlying anatomy of the condition

Muscular injuries. Muscle strains in hyperextension injuries of the neck involve the flexors of the head such as the sternocleidomastoid and rectus capitis anterior. Other flexors of the neck often injured are the longus colli and intertransverse muscles. Both groups of muscles lie along the anterior and anterolateral surfaces of the cervical spine and are overstretched in hyperextension. The damage ranges in severity from minor tears of a few muscle fibers to partial or total avulsion (traumatic separation) of the muscular attachments to the cervical spine. These injuries have been observed experimentally in anesthetized monkeys as well as clinically at the time of surgery or autopsy.

Ligamentous injuries. Ligamentous sprains are the mildest form of neck injuries. What is a sprain? A sprain denotes a ligamentous injury with stretching of some of the fibers and tearing of others but with preservation of the continuity of the ligament. Which ligament connecting the vertebral bodies would be most likely to be sprained in forceful hyperextension of the neck, and which in the opposite trauma of hyperflexion?

The thick anterior longitudinal ligament is a broad band that extends along the anterior surface of the vertebral column from the atlas to the front of the sacrum. While its more superficial fibers bridge several vertebrae, its deeper portions extend from one vertebral body to the next. It is particularly these deeper portions of the ligament that may be stretched or torn in hyperextension injuries (Fig. 2).

Hyperflexion injuries may expose the posterior longitudinal ligament to undue traction. The posterior longitudinal ligament likewise extends over all vertebrae from the neck to the sacrum with its superficial fibers crossing several vertebrae and its deeper portions connecting adjacent vertebrae. The posterior longitudinal ligament attaches to the posterior aspect of the vertebral bodies in front of the spinal cord and checks extreme flexion. In this function it is assisted by the ligamenta flava, which connect the laminar portions of the vertebral arches, and the interspinal and supraspinal ligaments. The latter are particularly well developed in the neck as the so-called ligamentum nuchae which in man forms a fibrous, intermuscular septum in the midline by attaching to the bifid spinous processes. The posterior longitudinal ligament and the ligamentum flavum may be stretched or torn in hyperflexion as result of a front-end collision.

Note: The reader is advised to supply himself with two or more adjacent cervical vertebrae, to locate the anatomical structures in their proper relationship. As a substitute, the use of an anatomical atlas is recommended.

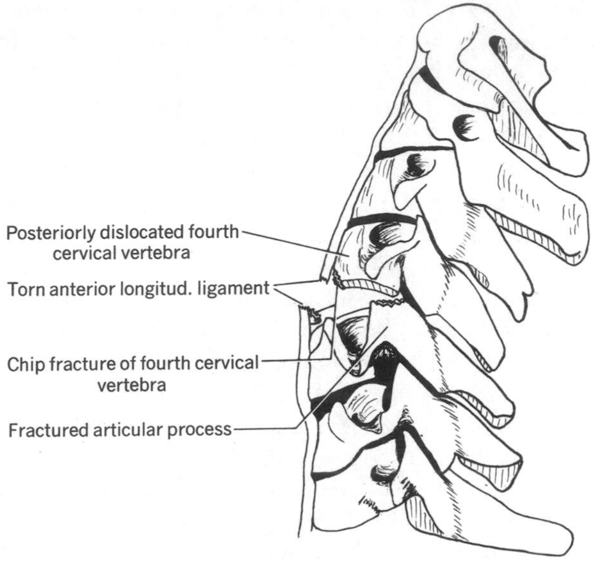

Figure 2—Extensive hyperextension injury with tearing of the anterior longitudinal ligament, posterior dislocation of the fourth cervical vertebra with chip fracture of its body, and fracture of the articular process of the fifth cervical vertebra.

Disk injuries. Injury to the cervical disks in rear-end collisions, although often assumed, is apparently not too frequent and is not readily confirmed by objective means. Name the two parts of an intervertebral disk and give the characteristic features of each portion. The outer ring, the anulus fibrosus, consists of concentric layers of collagenous fiber bundles, which by their arrangement are able to withstand strains. The centrally located nucleus pulposus consists of a soft, highly elastic, compressible, semi-gelatinous mass with high water content. It acts as a shock absorber.

How does uneven height of a given disk contribute to the normal cervical lordosis? The cervical disks are thicker anteriorly than posteriorly, and thus are responsible for the forward convex curvature of the cervical spine. Degenerative changes due to chronic trauma and age predispose the anulus fibrosus to rupture under severe compression and the nucleus pulposus to prolapse or herniate. This is particularly apt to occur in the neck at the level of the disks between cervical vertebrae five and six and vertebrae seven and eight.

Spinal nerve and cord involvement. Keeping in mind that the intervertebral disk forms part of the anterior boundary of the intervertebral foramen, in what direction would the protrusion of a damaged anulus or a herniated nucleus pulposus have to occur to compress a cervical nerve passing through this foramen? A posterolateral protrusion of the disk has this effect and explains the occurrence of nerve root symptoms such as shoulder pain and paresthesias (burning and tingling) in the affected dermatomes, perceived as far distally as the fingers in involvement of C6 and C7. The commonly observed reflex spasm of the neck muscles with straightening of the normal curvature of the spine is another effect of nerve or nerve root irritation. Most serious is a protrusion of the disk in, or close to, the midline, leading to cervical cord compression.

Vertebral injuries and dislocation. There is a gradual transition in severity from the relatively harmless and common stretching of the anterior longitudinal ligament to its rupture, to wrenching and displacement of the disks, and chip fracture of the anterior-inferior corners of the vertebral bodies (Fig. 2). If the trauma is more destructive, the articular processes of the vertebrae may also fracture, and the upper part of the cervical spinal column may be dislocated posteriorly with pressure on and damage of the cord. In these cases, open reduction by means of surgery is often required to remove pressure on the cord.

The intervertebral foramina and synovial joints. The intervertebral foramina in the cervical region have been called the "crossroads of neurological symptomatology." They are short canals which contain the ventral and dorsal roots and their spinal ganglia within a meningeal sleeve, the recurrent meningeal nerves, the spinal arteries, and venous plexuses, all embedded in fat and connective tissue. The venous plexuses connecting the internal and external spinal veins allow blood to be expelled in movements of the cervical column, thus cushioning and protecting the nerve structures against pressure. The same holds true for the fat which is semifluid at body temperature.

Immediately posterior to the intervertebral foramina are the superior and inferior articular processes of adjacent vertebrae forming synovial joints, which are surrounded by a joint capsule (Fig. 1). Synovial joints are subject to many inflammatory arthritic and degenerative diseases which frequently lead to changes in joint configuration by narrowing of the articulations, thickening of the joint capsule, and bony spur formation (bone proliferation). These changes result in alterations in spatial relationship and encroachment on the intervertebral foramina, and in hyperextension trauma expose the sensitive nerve structures within the foramina to stretching over preexisting abnormal bone formation. The presence of bony spurs adjacent to the intervertebral foramina between C4 and C5 was mentioned in our case and could partly explain the symptoms of our patient.

Occasionally, a nerve root or parts of a nerve root may be caught, pincer-like, between deformed articular facets. It was mentioned previously that the intervertebral disks are an immediate anterior boundary of the intervertebral foramina and that protrusion of these disks as result of trauma may explain the signs and symptoms of nerve involvement in disk degeneration (Fig. 1).

Uncovertebral joints. Another anatomical arrangement, typical only of the cervical area, has been the subject of extensive discussion in the clinical literature, although often ignored in anatomical texts, i.e. the uncovertebral joints (lateral interbody joints, joints of Luschka). Although not true synovial joints, but apparently the result of degenerative prossesses starting in the cervical disks in childhood and adolescence, they give the appearance of joints. They are formed by the upward lip-like projection on the superior surface of the cervical vertebral bodies (uncinate process) and corresponding beveled grooves on the inferiorlateral surface of the overlying vertebrae. These bony areas are covered with cartilage and surrounded by a synovia-like capsule. The presence of these joints predisposes to disk collapse and arthritic changes with bone proliferation. They are part of the anterior boundary of the intervertebral foramina and lie in close relationship to their nerve root contents (Fig. 1). Again, as with other degenerative and proliferative joint changes, superimposed trauma on these joints leads to or aggravates the clinical condition of nerve root compression.

In summary then, we have the nerve structures within the intervertebral foramina bounded anteriorly and anterolaterally by the cartilaginous joints between vertebral bodies and incorporating the intervertebral disks; by the uncovertebral joints anterolaterally; and posteriorly by the intervertebral synovial joints. All these articulations alter their configuration during flexion, extension, and torsion of the cervical spine and thereby encroach on the intervertebral foramina and their contents. This is particularly true in hyperextension and the more so, if the joints are already deformed by degenerative or proliferative bone changes. It is easily realized that the emergence of spinal nerves from the spinal canal through foramina that are bounded anteriorly and posteriorly by movable joints is conducive to injury of these nerves. How does this compare with the emergence of the cranial nerves from the skull? Here the nerves leave the cranial cavity through bony foramina that are not exposed to changing contours of their boundaries. What spinal nerves have an arrangement similar to that of the cranial nerves? The sacral nerves leave the spinal canal through sacral foramina bounded by solid bone.

Vertebral artery injury. A final and sometimes quite serious complication of hyperextension injury is compression of the vertebral artery as it runs through the neck. What is its course in the neck? It is the first branch of the subclavian artery and ascends through the transverse foramina of the cervical vertebrae starting with C6 and leaving through the transverse foramen of the atlas, to enter the cranial cavity through the greater occipital foramen. In addition to giving off spinal branches, it joins with its partner of the opposite side to form the basilar artery, which supplies the posterior portion of the brain. As the vertebral artery passes through the transverse foramina it lies in front of the emerging nerve roots. Hyper-extension injury may traumatize the artery, particularly if its walls have become arteriosclerotic and rigid and may lead to vascular insufficiency of the posterior portions of the brain. Bizarre clinical pictures, such as vertigo, ataxia (loss of muscular coordination), disturbances of vision and hearing, and temporary loss of consciousness may result. Some of these symptoms are caused by vasospasm as result of the trauma, which may be transitory; others, more lasting, may occur due to direct injury to the artery. It should not be overlooked that the vertebral artery is surrounded by a sympathetic plexus and that some of the previously mentioned clinical manifestations may be caused by its irritation.

Fortunately for our patient, her symptoms were transitory. They can probably be explained by a ligamentous sprain with resulting muscle spasm and some temporary injury to the cervical nerves which may have been stretched over existing bone proliferations at levels C4 and C5.

Body Wall and Back

8 Cancer of the Breast

A 51-year-old housewife comes to the clinic because one month earlier she had noticed a lump in her right breast. Since then she has had occasional dull aches in her breast. She has applied iodine but received no benefit. Her personal physician diagnosed cancer. She has always been in good health, never having consulted a physician except at childbirths, of which she has had three. She reached her menopause eight years ago.

EXAMINATION

The patient is a rugged woman apparently in the best of health. As she sits in the chair the right nipple is a good half inch higher than the left. The upper outer quadrant of the right breast contains a reddened area two inches in diameter. The borders of this shade gradually into the surrounding skin. This area is flatter in contour than the same area of the left breast, and the skin over the area seems dimpled. As the patient is turned from side to side and bent forward, the right breast remains rigid and does not respond to the action of gravity, as does the other breast. The axilla of the right side seems fuller than on the left.

On palpation the reddened area described above is found to be hard, board-like, and the whole upper outer quadrant of

The history and clinical findings of this case study, greatly modified, are taken from a classical collection of case studies, A. E. Hertzler's Clinical Surgery by Case Histories, St. Louis, C. V. Mosby Company, 1921, vol. 1, 317.

the breast appears as a solid mass. The whole breast moves freely over the pectoral fascia, but the skin in the involved quadrant is firmly fixed and has the hard, rough corrugated feel of an orange peel. The right nipple is retracted and fixed and does not respond to traction, whereas the left does. The right axilla is occupied by a solid mass in which no separate tumor masses can be made out, but the whole mass is freely movable on the surrounding tissues. There are no supraclavicular nodes palpable. Both this mass in the breast and the tumor in the axilla are sensitive to firm pressure. All other examinations are negative.

DIAGNOSIS

Cancer of the breast with axillary metastases.

THERAPY

A radical breast operation was done with removal of breast, pectoralis major and pectoralis minor muscles, of axillary lymph nodes and axillary fat. The tributaries of the axillary vein in the operative field were also removed, but the long thoracic and the thoracodorsal nerves were identified and preserved. Microscopic study of the breast and axillary nodes confirmed the diagnosis of cancer.

FURTHER COURSE

The patient had an uneventful postoperative recovery but complained of some swelling of her arm, which was treated with physiotherapy. Six months later she had a recurrence in the axilla and died of lung metastasis nine months after surgery.

DISCUSSION

The physical findings of a large mass in the right breast, the dimpling and fixation of the skin in the involved quadrant,

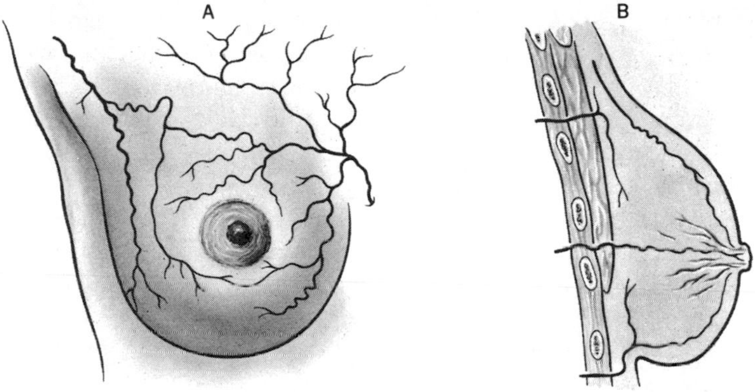

Figure 1A.—Front view of arterial supply to breast showing medial and lateral mammary branches from the internal thoracic and lateral thoracic arteries respectively. Other lateral mammary branches originate from the thoracoacromial and intercostal arteries. Medial and lateral mammary branches communicate around the nipple. B.—Parasagittal section of breast showing in addition to the arteries visualized in Figure 1A, deep (perforating) mammary branches passing through the intercostal spaces.

the retracted and fixed nipple, and the mass in the axilla leave no doubt as to the advanced stage of the cancer.

Anatomical signs of spread in breast cancer

What is the reason for the reddening of the skin in the area of the cancer? The reddening of the skin over the tumor is due to increased flow of blood to and from the area. The blood supply to the breast is derived mainly from the internal thoracic, the lateral thoracic, the posterior intercostal, and the thoraco-acromial arteries, which give off medial, lateral, and deep (perforating) mammary arteries (Fig. 1, A and B). Veins essentially follow the course of the arteries.

How do you explain the fixation of the skin to the tumor and the orange-peel-like appearance of the skin? The dimpling and fixation of the skin to the tumor implies cancerous invasion of the suspensory ligaments (of Cooper) which anchor the gland to the skin (Fig. 2). The orange-peel-like appearance of the skin indicates cancerous obstruction of the lymphatics draining the skin, while the hair follicles and cutaneous glands, being more firmly attached to the subcutaneous tissue, withstand the expansion caused by lymph blockage and therefore appear as pits or depressions (Fig. 2).

What does the elevation, retraction, and fixation of the nipple mean in anatomical terms? The elevation, retraction, and fixation of the right nipple is explained on the basis of cancerous involvement and subsequent scarring of the lactiferous ducts (Fig. 2).

How do you explain the mass in the axilla? The axillary tumor is a typical sign of cancerous spread to the axillary lymph nodes, the site of the principal lymph drainage of the breast.

Identify the lymph nodes in the axillary fossa where a cluster of cancer cells (embolus) might be arrested after it has become detached from the primary cancer of the breast.

The axillary lymph nodes

The term "axillary nodes" applies to a large aggregation of nodes located within the pyramidal space of the axilla. Their separation into individual groups is somewhat artificial but facilitates the understanding of regional lymphatic drainage and helps to clarify the location of the nodes. However, it should be understood that the axillary nodes are subject to great variations in location, size, and number and that the groups have a rich system of interconnecting anastomoses.

There are all together five groups, the first three of which can be regarded as peripheral outposts, while the other two are more centrally located within the axillary fossa and toward its apex. These groups of nodes are: (1) the lateral set along the upper part of the humerus in the medial bicipital groove in relation to the axillary vein; (2) the subscapular set following the posterior axillary fold along the lateral border of the scapula in relation to the thoracodorsal and subscapular veins;

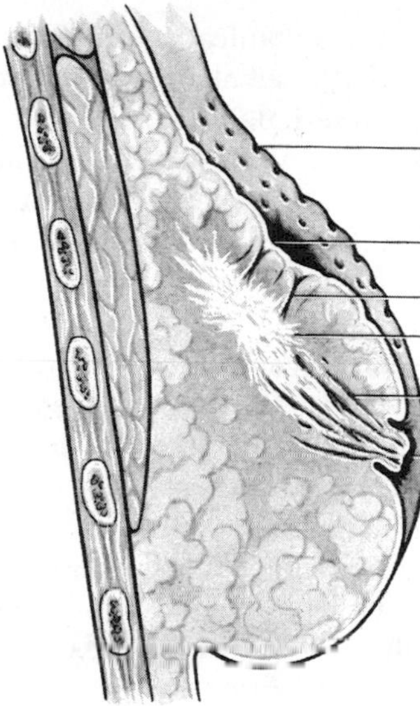

Figure 2—Dimpling and orange-peel-like appearance of the skin and retraction and elevation of the nipple, signs of cancerous spread to suspensory ligaments of the breast, obstruction of the cutaneous lymphatics, and involvement of the lactiferous ducts.

(3) the pectoral set beneath the anterior axillary fold in relation to the lateral thoracic veins; (4) the central set formed by rather large and fairly numerous nodes in the fat of the axilla which receives the preceding three outlying groups; (5) the apical set behind the costocoracoid membrane in relation to the more proximal part of the axillary vein. It receives the efferent vessels from all other groups.

The axillary nodes, taken as a whole, receive two streams of lymph, one coming from the upper extremity, the other from the adjacent thoracic wall, particularly from the breast. The two currents meet and fuse within the central and apical chains. While the lymph from the arm drains into the outlying lateral nodes, the lymph from the breast is filtered mainly by the pectoral nodes in which the lymph trunks from the breast terminate. The efferent vessels from the pectoral nodes go to the central set which drains into the apical nodes. From there the lymph empties by way of the subclavian trunk into the junction of the subclavian and internal jugular veins, or it may terminate on the right side in the right lymphatic duct and on the left side in the thoracic duct, being in part filtered through the supraclavicular (inferior deep cervical) nodes.

Thus, we have the following lymph nodes interposed in the pathway of cancerous emboli from the breast before they reach the venous bloodstream: pectoral, central, and apical (supraclavicular). Shortcuts that bypass one, two, or even three of the more peripheral lymphatic stations may occur; hence direct drainage from the breast into the central or apical or even the supraclavicular set can take place. In the latter case, we have the clinical picture of enlarged supraclavicular nodes without involvement of the axillary nodes, a condition which most surgeons regard as inoperable. A direct lymphatic channel from the deeper superior portions of the mammary gland to the apical nodes is well known. It passes around the inferior border or through the substance of the pectoralis major and ascends on the surface of or deep to the pectoralis minor to the apical nodes. Small interpectoral nodes may be interposed in this pathway. The possible presence of this channel explains the need for removal of both pectoral muscles in radical mastectomy. As stated before, anastomoses between the outlying pectoral, lateral, and subscapular chains are present, so that the latter two may likewise, though rarely, be affected in cancer of the breast.

Accessory lymphatic channels

Additional lymph vessels connect the breast and particularly its medial half with the sternal nodes. These vessels traverse the pectoralis major and internal intercostal muscles and follow in their course the perforating branches of the internal thoracic vessels. They terminate in nodes located in the upper intercostal spaces in relation to the internal thoracic vessels close to the lateral margin of the sternum. These nodes tend to disappear in old age. Their efferents go to the supraclavicular nodes and lymph trunks in the neck. A few surgeons have devised a supraradical resection of the breast that includes removal of the sternal nodes. Improvement of results by this surgical approach is questionable. Direct lymphatic connections to the opposite breast and opposite axilla have also been postulated on the basis of clinical evidence in breast cancer.

In this discussion on lymphatic drainage of the breast and lymphatic spread of cancerous emboli, it must be realized that obstruction of the normal lymph current by metastatic growth in the lymph nodes may lead to reversal of the lymph flow and to involvement of lymph nodes in atypical locations, e.g. the inguinal region.

Vulnerable nerves in mastectomy

What important motor nerves should be identified and preserved, as was done in our case? What muscles do they supply and what is the effect of injury to either nerve? The long thoracic nerve supplies the important serratus anterior, whose paralysis results in "winged" scapula. Injury to the thoracodorsal nerve leads to loss of function of the latissimus dorsi and therefore to difficulties in extension, adduction, and medial rotation of the humerus. The latter two motions are already compromised by the removal of the pectoralis major.

Anatomy of edema

What is the cause of the postoperative swelling (edema) of the upper extremity? It is presumed to be due to a combination of lymphatic and venous obstruction. The former results from the severance and removal of most of the lymphatic channels that drain the arm; the latter is caused by the frequently occurring thrombosis of the axillary vein, which is the consequence of the necessary surgical handling and endothelial injury of the vein. Delicate dissection at the time of surgery with massage and physiotherapy postoperatively will alleviate the swelling.

PROGNOSIS

With what stage of the cancer are we dealing in this case? The attachment of the skin to the tumor, the reddening and swelling of the skin over the tumor, the fixation of the nipple, and particularly the pronounced axillary involvement are all signs of a fairly advanced cancer of the breast.

What anatomical findings are favorable to the patient? The location in the upper outer quadrant of the breast is the most common and, according to many authors, the most favorable site of cancer. The mobility of the breast over the pectoral fascia is a sign of non-involvement of the underlying fascia and muscle and is therefore advantageous to the patient. The absence of palpable supraclavicular lymph nodes is also a relatively favorable sign.

In view of the short history and the relatively advanced state of the breast cancer, the prognosis on admission would have to be very guarded in spite of the technical operability of the tumor and its axillary metastasis.

9 Indirect Inguinal Hernia

A 10-year-old boy comes to the outpatient department with the complaint that from time to time, particularly when he stands or strains, a "bulge" appears in his right groin. Off and on there is moderate pain in this area which is increased by lifting a heavy object or by pushing a cart.

EXAMINATION

On inspection in the upright position, a bulge of walnut size is noticeable in the right inguinal area which increases in volume on coughing or nose blowing. On palpation the swelling seems to extend upward into the inguinal canal. However, its upper end cannot be felt. With the patient in the horizontal position the lump disappears. When the examiner invaginates the skin of the scrotum and inserts his little finger into the superficial inguinal ring, he feels a definite impact on coughing. On straining the bulge becomes again demonstrable, also in the horizontal position. It can be reduced by the examiner and when after reduction his fingers are pressed firmly over the area of the internal inguinal ring, the mass does not descend into the inguinal canal. Examination of the left side does not reveal any abnormality.

DIAGNOSIS

Right-sided, complete, reducible, indirect inguinal hernia.

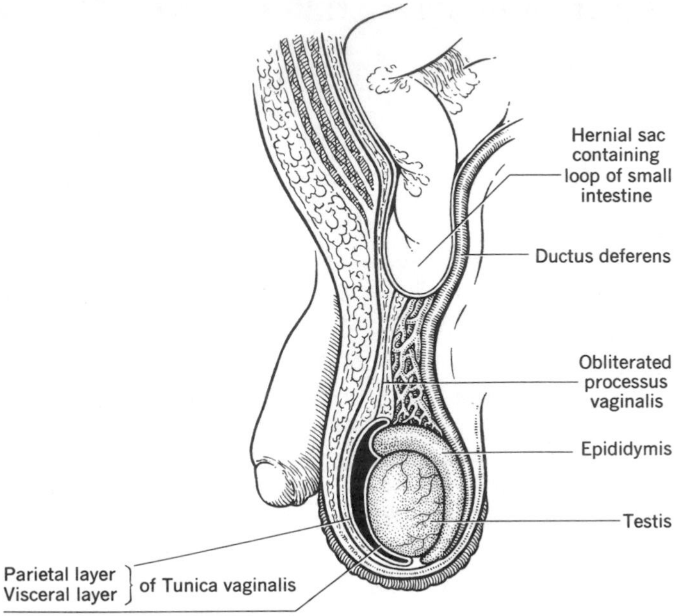

Figure 1 shows section through an indirect, inguinal hernia with the hernial sac containing a loop of small intestine. Notice partial obliteration of processus vaginalis.

THERAPY AND FURTHER COURSE

The treatment of choice of inguinal hernia in a boy ten years of age is surgery, since spontaneous obliteration of the hernial sac at this age does not occur. The patient is operated one week later.

Under general anesthesia, the skin and superficial fascia are divided by an incision above and parallel to the inguinal ligament down to the aponeurosis of the external oblique muscle. Blood vessels encountered in the superficial fascia are clamped and ligated.

The inguinal canal is opened by incising the aponeurosis of the external oblique muscle. This incision extends the length of the canal and includes the superficial inguinal ring. The ilioinguinal nerve is identified and carefully displaced. Both portions of the divided external oblique are reflected by blunt dissection. With reflection of the anterior wall of the canal, the cord and hernial sac within the coverings of the cord are visualized. By blunt dissection the coverings of the cord are removed from the hernial sac and the sac isolated. The walls of the sac are then carefully incised without injury to its contents. The contents in this case consist of a loop of small intestine (Fig. 1). The intestine is gently replaced into the general peritoneal cavity. The sac is then separated by dissection from the structures of the cord which lie lateral and posterior to the sac. After the sac has been widely opened and carefully inspected for absence of any further contents, the sac is ligated at its proximal end and excised. The spermatic cord is replaced in its normal position and the divided portions of the external oblique aponeurosis, including the superficial inguinal ring, are reunited. The superficial fascia and skin incisions are closed in layers.

The patient is out of bed for short periods on the first postoperative day and leaves the hospital a week later. The mother is told to restrict physical activities of the boy for six weeks. On reexamination he shows no signs of recurrence and has no complaints.

DISCUSSION

We are dealing here with a complete, right-sided, reducible, indirect inguinal hernia. What is your definition of an indirect inguinal heria?

An indirect inguinal hernia is a hernia in which an out pouching of the peritoneal sac enters the inguinal canal at the deep inguinal ring, and if complete leaves it at the superficial inguinal ring. In other words, the hernial sac, formed by peritoneum and containing abdominal contents, takes the same course through the abdominal wall as the spermatic cord. Why is the term "indirect" applied to this type of inguinal hernia? An indirect inguinal hernia chooses an oblique and longer pathway through the abdominal wall than the direct type. The latter enters the abdominal wall directly posterior to the superficial ring and therefore penetrates the inguinal canal through its posterior wall medial to the deep ring.

What is the cause of indirect inguinal hernia? The predisposing factor essential to the development of an indirect inguinal hernia is the persistence of the processus vaginalis. Define this processus. It is a diverticulum or outpouching of the peritoneum which, during embryonal development, precedes the testis in its migration into the scrotum, evaginating before it all layers of the abdominal wall it encounters in its descent. While the lower portion of this peritoneal diverticulum remains patent as the tunica vaginalis testis, its upper part becomes obliterated. This obliteration normally takes place during the first postnatal year or even later, with the right side becoming occluded later than the left. This factor seems to explain the higher incidence of right-sided inguinal hernia. This is also the site of the hernia in our case.

Indirect inguinal hernia and inguinal canal

Can the presence of an open processus vaginalis be equated with an indirect inguinal hernia? A patent vaginal process, while predisposing to congenital inguinal hernia, is not at all identical with this clinical entity, since the latter implies the protrusion of a viscus or part of a viscus through the deep inguinal ring into this preformed sac. What is the deep inguinal ring and at what point is it projected on the surface of the anterior abdominal wall? Simply and somewhat inaccurately defined, the deep ring is an opening in the transversalis fascia. Actually it is the site where the transversalis fascia is continued as an attenuated outpouching over the spermatic cord, forming its innermost sheath, that is, the internal spermatic fascia. The deep ring is located about one-half inch above the midpoint of the inguinal ligament. Remember that the inguinal ligament does not extend to the midline, but only as far as the pubic tubercle.

Since the normal inguinal canal represents a weakness of

the anterior abdominal wall, what counteracts the formation of a hernia even in the presence of a partially or totally open processus vaginalis? The obliquity of the canal constitutes a natural obstacle to the formation of a hernia. Increase in intra-abdominal pressure, such as takes place in coughing, straining, nose blowing, or crying, actually forces the walls of the canal closer together. In addition, a shutter-like mechanism at the deep ring narrows its opening when the internal oblique and transversus muscles contract. If the cremaster muscle is well developed, a recoil-like action of its fibers pulls the cord like a plug toward the internal ring.

Herniation through the deep inguinal ring into the open processus vaginalis occurs only after the ring has become wide enough to permit some content of the peritoneal cavity to extrude through the ring into the canal in conjunction with the spermatic cord. What is the relation of the hernial sac to the structures of the cord? The hernial sac lies within the substance of the cord, ensheathed by the internal spermatic fascia and cremaster muscle and fascia. These form the coverings of the cord within the inguinal canal. The ductus deferens lies immediately posterior to the sac to which it is joined by areolar tissue, the latter being a derivative of the extraperitoneal connective tissue (Fig. 2).

What structure has to be incised to open the anterior wall of the inguinal canal and make the cord and hernia visible? What forms the superficial inguinal ring, which is likewise cut by this incision, and where is it located? The aponeurosis of the external oblique forms the anterior wall of the inguinal canal, reinforced laterally on its deep aspect by muscle fibers of the internal oblique arising from the inguinal ligament and the iliac fascia. The superficial inguinal ring is a triangular gap in the aponeurosis of the external oblique. To be specific, it is the site where the aponeurosis of the external oblique is attenuated to be continued over the cord and the sac of a complete hernia as its outermost sheath, the external spermatic fascia. The superficial ring lies cranial and lateral to the pubic crest. Its lateral (inferior) crus coincides with the attachment

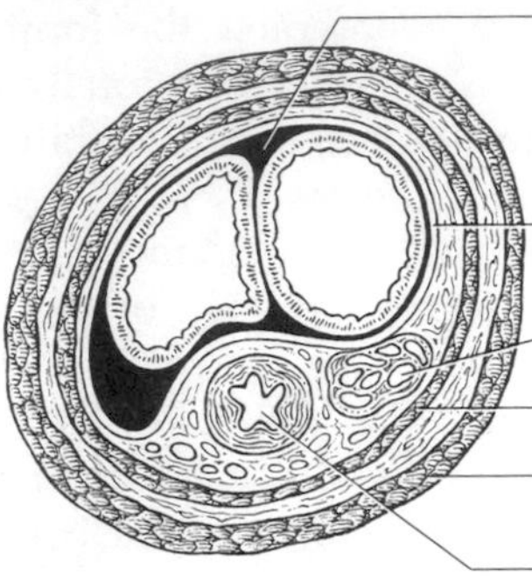

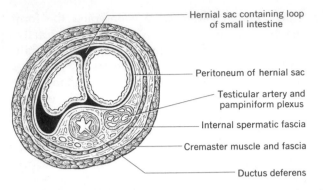

Figure 2 shows cross-section through spermatic cord and hernial sac containing a loop of small intestine. Notice that the hernia forms part of the contents of the cord and is surrounded by its coverings. Also notice the typical location of the sac in front of the ductus deferens.

of the inguinal ligament to the pubic tubercle, while its medial (superior) crus inserts on the pubic bone as part of the external oblique.

In children with large herniae and in adults, an additional step in the surgery of indirect inguinal hernia commonly is the suturing of the falx inguinalis to the inguinal ligament. This procedure strengthens the posterior wall of the inguinal canal. What is the falx inguinalis? It is a part of the lower arching fibers of the internal oblique and transversus muscles that insert into the pubic bone. The falx is nonuniform in composition, being variably muscular, tendinous, or fascial in character in different subjects. This is also the reason why its synonym "conjoined tendon" has become obsolete, since the two muscles may neither join nor be tendinous in this area.

Anatomy of surgical complications

Endangered Nerves—During surgery in our case, as in every case of inguinal hernia, attention is paid to what nerve? The ilioinguinal nerve is particularly endangered, since it lies in the operative field and passes through the superficial inguinal ring. It supplies the skin of the anterior portion of the scrotum and the adjacent region of the thigh with sensory fibers. If it is divided within the canal, numbness of the scrotum and inner aspect of the thigh results. If it is included in a suture or embedded in scar tissue, postoperative neuritic pain will ensue.

Do the ilioinguinal and the more cranially located iliohypogastric nerves, both of which lie in the operative area, carry motor fibers? At a more cranial level both of these nerves have motor components which supply the lowermost portions of the internal oblique and transverse muscles. Section of these nerves at this level would interfere with the nerve supply to the muscular portions mentioned and thus lead to weakness of the posterior wall of the inguinal canal. This might result in recurrence of the hernia.

Endangered Blood Vessels—Postoperative hemorrhage is probably the most common complication of inguinal hernia. What blood vessels are encountered in this operation in the deep part of the subcutaneous tissue? Of what vessels are they branches? The superficial epigastric artery and vein, ascending in a medial direction across the midportion of the inguinal ligament, are divided and ligated in this operation. They are branches of the femoral artery and great saphenous vein respectively. The superficial external pudendal artery and vein, which are branches of the same vessels, may also be encountered.

What major vessel lies in close relation to the deep ring whose injury may cause serious hemorrhage? The inferior epigastric artery, one of the two main branches of the external iliac artery, may be inadvertently cut. If it is not ligated after such an accident, severe bleeding will result. What is the relation of the inferior epigastric artery to the internal ring, and therefore to the point of entrance, of an indirect inguinal hernia into the abdominal wall?

It lies medial to the internal ring, but it forms the lateral boundary of the inguinal triangle, which is the site of entrance of a direct inguinal hernia.

Injury to Ductus Deferens and Bladder—Another undesirable accident in herniorrhaphy is inadvertent cutting of the ductus deferens when the hernial sac is freed from its environment. In what relationship to the sac does the ductus deferens lie and how can you identify it by palpation? It lies immediately posterior to the sac and can be recognized by its hard and whipcord-like feel when it is rolled between thumb and index finger. Division of the ductus deferens will result in sterility on this side. An attempt at reuniting the divided ends should be made. Damage to the testicular artery should likewise be avoided since it may also result in infertility on one side.

What organ situated in the lesser pelvis in the adult lies in a more abdominal location in the infant and may be in close proximity to the internal ring? In infants the bladder may overlap the internal ring and may be inadvertently incised in herniorrhaphy. This complication, while not harmless, can be taken care of by suture closure if recognized during surgery.

Incarceration and Strangulation—Define the complications of incarceration and strangulation of a hernia. In incarceration the hernia is irreducible and there is obstruction to the passage of intestinal contents in the herniated portion of the intestine, but the blood supply to the viscus remains unaffected. In strangulated hernia the blood supply and lymph drainage of the herniated viscus are impaired or occluded. Depending on the degree of vascular occlusion, the intestinal loop will lose its viability within hours unless the hernia is attended to immediately.

10 Prolapse of Intervertebral Disk

A 43-year-old college professor tried to push his car, which was caught in a snowdrift, and immediately suffered sudden and severe pain in the lower back. He felt as if something had "snapped" in the lower part of his spine. Later his pain extended down the posterior aspect of his right thigh and leg. He also noticed some numbness and tingling over the lateral part of his right leg, foot, and little toe. He reported that for several years past he has had episodes of "lame back," particularly after lifting heavy objects from a stooping position.

EXAMINATION

On examination the patient complains of a dull ache in the lower back, which is aggravated by straining and coughing. There is a diminution in the spinal lumbar curve and a tilt of the trunk to the left side. Due to pain there is marked limitation of movement in the lumbar spinal column. Raising of his right extended leg is quite painful. On further examination there is tenderness to palpation along the course of the sciatic nerve in the right thigh. There is some weakness in plantar flexion of his right foot as well as some loss of sensory perception over the dorsal side of the right fourth and fifth toes.

DIAGNOSIS

Rupture of the intervertebral disk between the fifth lumbar

and first sacral vertebrae with protrusion of the nucleus pulposus and nerve root involvement of the first sacral nerve.

THERAPY AND FURTHER COURSE

Under conservative treatment and bed rest on a reinforced hard mattress, physiotherapy, and traction, the patient improved sufficiently to be discharged from the hospital.

DISCUSSION

The combination of low back pain and pain along the course of the sciatic nerve aggravated by straining is rather typical of a disk lesion. What is the function of the intervertebral disk and what are its two components? The intervertebral disks act as shock absorbers and consist of an outer firm fibrocartilaginous ring, the anulus fibrosus, and an inner softer, more pliable, gelatinous center, the nucleus pulposus. Chronic trauma, particularly in the middle-aged or older patient with degenerative changes in the intervertebral disk, leads to a posterior tear in the anulus fibrosus, at the site of greatest mechanical stress. A later consequence, particularly in conjunction with further acute or chronic trauma, is protrusion or herniation of the nucleus pulposus into the spinal canal. Usually the herniation takes place to one side of the midline because of the ligamentous reinforcement in the midline. What is the name of the ligament that runs along the posterior aspect of the bodies of the vertebrae from the atlas to the sacrum and is intimately blended with the disks? The posterior longitudinal ligament attaches to the occiput above and extends all the way down into the sacral canal. It narrows behind each vertebral body but broadens over the disks.

The "snap" that the patient felt may have been caused by the anular tear, with partial expulsion of the nucleus pulposus. The lower lumbar disks are the most common sites of herniation, this being one of the most flexible areas of the spinal column. The disappearance of the normal lumbar concavity or lordosis is due to exaggerated contraction of what group of muscles responsible for motions of the spinal column? The disappearance of the normal lumbar concavity is due to exaggerated contraction of the flexors. Pain in disk lesions is increased by extension and reduced by flexion of the lumbar spine. What are its main flexors? The chief flexors of the lumbar spinal column are the rectus abdominis and the iliopsoas muscles.

Cauda equina and subarachnoid space

Is the spinal cord subjected to pressure at the level indicated? What is the lowest extent of the cord in terms of vertebral level? Is the area involved within the extent of the subarachnoidal space? Remember that the cord in the adult ends approximately at the level of the second lumbar and the subarachnoid space at the level of the second sacral vertebra. What are the contents of the thecal (meningeal) sac below the level of the cord? The contents of the thecal sac caudal to the conus medullaris are cerebrospinal fluid, the cauda equina, and the filum terminale. Does the cauda equina consist of spinal nerves or nerve roots? The cauda equina consists of nerve roots which continue downward in the spinal canal within the meningeal sac, approximately to the level of emergence from their intervertebral foramina, and are covered by meningeal sleeves as far as the spinal ganglia. Here the meningeal membranes are continuous with the epineurium.

Posterolateral herniation of the nucleus pulposus may readily impinge upon the nerve roots within the spinal canal as they course diagonally downward toward their exit (Fig. 1). The prolapse is particularly apt to compress the roots of the next lower spinal nerve. Thus herniation of the disk between the fifth lumbar and the first sacral vertebra involves most commonly the roots of the first sacral nerve, as in the case presented here (Figs. 1 and 2).

How do you explain the aggravation of pain by straining and coughing? These actions by increasing the intravenous pressure also increase the pressure of the cerebrospinal fluid, which adds to the pressure on the involved nerve root. On the

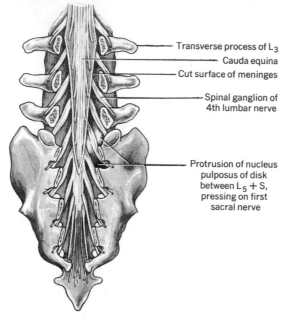

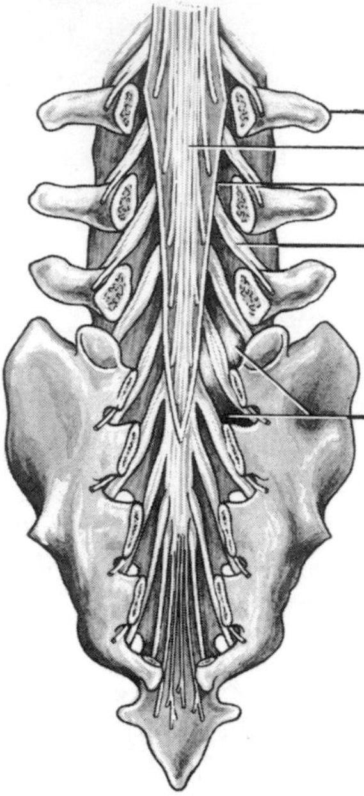

Figure 1—Vertebral arches have been removed and spinal canal has been exposed. The dura and arachnoid have been cut and reflected. The oblique course of spinal nerves is shown. Observe prolapsed nucleus pulposus pressing on first sacral nerve and ganglion.

other hand, listing of the trunk away from the compressed root decreases the pressure on the root and lessens the pain.

Sciatic nerve and its roots

The roots of the first sacral nerve represent one of the important components of the sciatic nerve. What are its other components? The sciatic nerve takes origin from the fourth and fifth lumbar and the first three sacral nerves. Raising of the extended leg of the patient in the recumbent position puts the sciatic nerve on the stretch and is painful in cases of sciatic nerve root compression, as is direct pressure on the sciatic

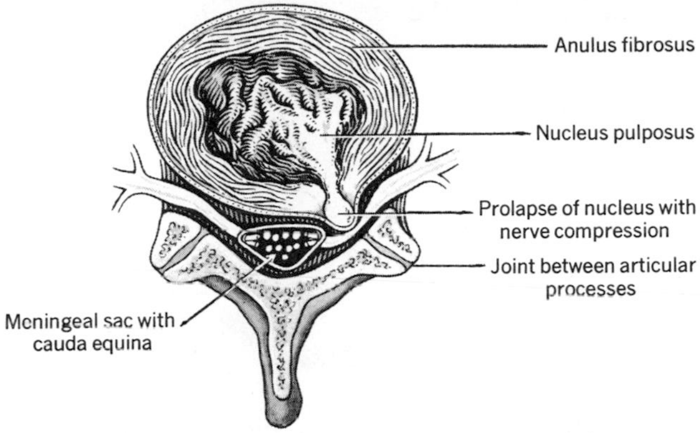

Figure 2—Cross-section of intervertebral disk and spinal canal. Observe ruptured anulus fibrosus with posterior protrusion of nucleus pulposus and compression of spinal nerve on the right.

nerve itself in its course along the thigh. Where in the thigh can you readily subject the nerve to pressure? Remember that the nerve runs almost vertically down the thigh midway between the great trochanter and the ischial tuberosity.

Weakness of plantar flexion of the right foot is a sign of involvement of the motor root of the first sacral nerve. Clinical experience shows that the branch of the tibial nerve supplying the main plantar flexor, the gastrocnemius muscle, does not contain fibers from all five motor roots of the sciatic nerve but mainly fibers from the first and second sacral nerve. The sensory area of the skin supplied by the first sacral nerve (dermatome) is somewhat variable and is under dispute. The most typical area of disturbed sensation in involvement of the first sacral nerve comprises the lateral aspect of the leg below the knee and the lateralmost toes. These are also the areas involved in this patient.

11 Lumbar Puncture

A 15-year-old boy is referred to the hospital by his family physician with symptoms of sneezing and coughing, severe headache, stiffness of the neck, and high fever.

EXAMINATION

On physical examination the boy, although in good nutritional state, appears to be quite ill and restless. He is drowsy and responds to questions rather hesitatingly, as if he has difficulty orienting himself. His reaction to physical stimuli is slow. His temperature is 104° and his pulse rate is accelerated. He displays all signs of an upper respiratory infection, but the lungs are clear. He complains of severe headache, which extends into the neck and is symmetrical on both sides of the head. On forward bending of the head and neck (flexion), the neck appears rather stiff. This movement is painful and is actively resisted by the patient.

Neurologic examination does not reveal any specific defect in the central nervous system. Functions of cranial and spinal nerves are intact. Examination of the fundus of the eye (eye grounds) with the ophthalmoscope shows the interior of the eye to be normal; especially is there no swelling of the optic discs, the site of entrance of the optic nerve into the eyeball. Increased intracranial pressure is therefore unlikely. In order to confirm or exclude the diagnosis of infectious meningitis, lumbar puncture is done. Although cerebral spinal fluid pressure is somewhat elevated, the fluid itself is clear, colorless and of normal protein and cell content. Consequently, infectious meningitis can be ruled out.

DIAGNOSIS

Febrile upper respiratory infection with meningeal irritation (meningismus).

THERAPY AND FURTHER COURSE

The patient is given antibiotic treatment to avoid spread of the infection to the lungs. Antipyretics and sedatives are prescribed against the fever, headache, and general discomfort. The fever is further reduced by frequent sponging with tap water and alcohol solution. Ice bags are applied to the patient's head.

During the next few days the patient continues to complain of headache, but his fever, general malaise, and upper respiratory symptoms gradually subside. The patient is discharged from the hospital after ten days. Follow up shows that he has completely recovered.

DISCUSSION

What is lumbar puncture (LP)?

Lumbar puncture is the tapping of the subarachnoid space in the lumbar region for the removal of cerebrospinal fluid (CSF) or for the introduction of drugs, such an antibiotics or steroids.

Lumbar puncture was introduced into our diagnostic and therapeutic armamentarium more than seventy-five years ago and has proved to have been of unforeseen value as a sensitive diagnostic procedure and therapeutic tool. Why should edema of the optic papilla, a sign of increased intracranial pressure, be excluded before LP can be undertaken? Sudden pressure reduction in the subarachnoid space by LP in the presence of elevated intracranial pressure may lead to herniation of parts of the cerebellum through the greater occipital foramen into the spinal canal or to prolapse of portions of the temporal lobe through the tentorial notch. The result in either case may be a most serious or fatal compression of vital portions of the brain.

Site of LP

What is the optimal site of LP? It is done in the lower part of the lumbar spinal column between vertebrae L3 and L4, or L4 and L5, generally to the exclusion of higher levels of the column. Is there an external landmark available for the proper site of entrance of the LP needle? A horizontal line connecting the highest points of the iliac crests, as seen from the posterior aspect, crosses the midline at about the level of the spinous process of L4. The adjacent interspinous spaces above or below are then chosen as the site of LP. Does the direction of the lumbar spinous processes facilitate entrance of the needle into the spinal canal? In the lumbar area there is a wide space between adjacent, horizontally directed spinous processes; this allows easy access to the spinal canal (Fig. 1). Is the same true in other areas of the vertebral column? Entrance into the canal between thoracic spinous processes is impossible since they are directed caudally and overlap each other, so that there is no area in the midline that is free of bone. What movement of the lumbar spinal column widens the space between adjacent spinous processes and is therefore used in positioning of the patient for LP? Maximal flexion of the spinal column (arching of the back) is applied either in the sitting or lateral horizontal position, with the knees of the patient drawn up as close to his chin as possible.

Lowest extent of the spinal cord in infant and adult

Why are more cranially located areas of the spinal column excluded as puncture sites? Obviously, tapping of the spinal cord with resulting injury to the central nervous system has to be avoided. The problem then focuses on the question: What is the lowest extent of the spinal cord in terms of vertebral

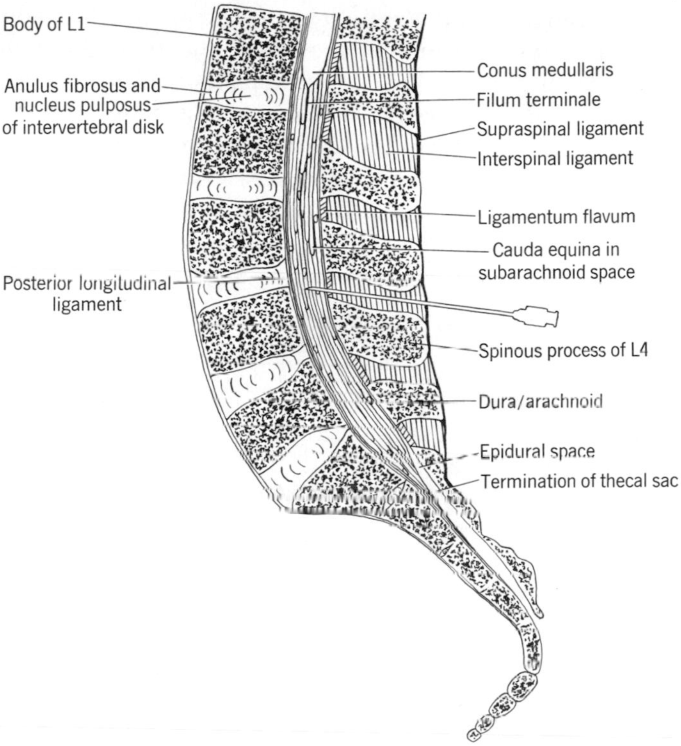

Figure 1—Midsagittal section through lumbar spinal column with spinal puncture needle in place between spinous processes of L3 and L4. Notice the slightly ascending direction of the needle. The needle has pierced three ligaments and the dura/arachnoid and is in the subarachnoid space.

landmarks? Is there any variation in the caudal extent of the cord? In the adult the lowest point of the cord is the conus medullaris. It is located at the lower border of the first lumbar or at the level of the body of the second lumbar vertebra. How do you explain that in the newborn and infant the terminal point of the cord is lower than the levels given for the adult? In the young fetus, the spinal cord extends through the whole length of the spinal canal down to the coccyx. As development progresses, the growth of the spinal cord does not keep pace with the longitudinal growth of the spinal column. Already at birth considerable discrepancy exists between the length of the cord and the column. At this date the cord ends at the inferior border of the third lumbar vertebra. Ultimately, the disproportion in length becomes even greater so that in the adult the end of the cord is generally two vertebrae higher, i.e. at the lower border of the first lumbar vertebra.

Subarachnoid space and Cauda equina

Between what meningeal layers is the spinal fluid located and what is the lowest extent of the meningeal (thecal) sac containing this fluid? The CSF fills the subarachnoid space between arachnoid and pia mater. The lowest extent of the subarachnoid space is at the level of the second sacral vertebra. Why then is spinal puncture not undertaken at lower levels than the typical sites, e.g. in the upper region of the sacrum? The solid bony mass of the posterior boundary of the sacral canal prevents entrance into this part of the subarachnoid space in the upper portion of the sacrum. Are there any nerve structures contained in the subarachnoid space that may be injured by LP below the level of the cord? The cauda equina (horse's tail) is a collection of spinal nerve roots (sensory and motor). They descend from the lowest part of the cord to their exit as spinal nerves through the lumbar intervertebral and sacral foramina. If students were asked approximately how many "hairs" make up the "horse's tail" just below the conus medullaris with a choice of 10, 20, 30, or 40 as an answer, the majority probably would choose 20, counting 4 lumbar, 5 sacral, and 1 coccygeal nerve on each side. Actually the answer is twice that many nerve structures since the spinal nerves have not yet formed and the contents of the subarachnoidal space are the ventral and dorsal roots rather than the nerves. The filum terminale which is essentially made up of pia mater should be added to the strands of hair of the horse's tail. Is injury to one of the nerve roots by the tip of the needle a danger in LP? If one of the roots is touched by the needle, it generally escapes injury, being easily displaced in the fluid medium. However, in case of contact with a sensory root the patient may perceive a shooting pain in his lower extremity on that side, and the needle should be withdrawn slightly.

Ligaments of the spine

What are the ligaments involved in LP? In the typical midline puncture three ligaments have to be traversed by the needle. Identify them. They are the supraspinal and interspinal ligaments and the ligamentum flavum (Fig. 1).

After the needle has pierced the skin and superficial fascia, these ligaments are encountered in the order given. The length of the needle has to be adjusted to the variable amount of fat in the subcutaneous tissue. The supraspinal ligaments connect the tips of the spinous processes; the interspinal ligaments join the superior and inferior borders of adjacent spinous processes and are fairly well developed in the lumbar area. The ligamenta flava are strong plate-like membranes, composed of yellow elastic fibers, that in the lumbar area may reach a thickness of 1 cm. They offer a noticeable resistance to the entering needle and their penetration is felt as a "snap" or "click." They run from the anterior-inferior border of the lamina of the higher vertebra to the posterior-superior aspect of the lamina of the adjacent lower vertebra. Thus, they cover the interlaminary space between two vertebrae, which on inspection of the skeleton and on the roentgenogram, appears to be quite large in this area. The ligamenta flava of the two sides meet in the midline at the root of the spinous process and fuse laterally with the capsules of the joints formed by the articular processes. They also blend posteriorly with the interspinal ligaments in the midline. It is the function of the ligamenta flava to assist the erector spinae muscle in sustaining the upright position. They are put on the stretch in flexion and their elastic pull helps to restore the upright (extended) posture. Since flexion is the position assumed by the patient in LP, the ligaments are stretched and more easily traversed by the needle than in the extended position of the body.

Epidural space and epidural anesthesia

Identify the potential space that the needle enters once LP has penetrated the ligamentum flavum. It is the epidural (peridural, extradural) space, which extends from the foramen magnum to the sacral hiatus and communicates through the intervertebral foramina with the space outside the spinal column. The epidural space surrounds the spinal meninges and separates the dura mater from the wall of the vertebral canal (Fig. 1). Its contents are the ventral and dorsal nerve roots, enveloped by their meningeal sleeve, and fatty and areolar tissue, in which a fair-sized vertebral plexus of veins, small arteries, and lymphatics are embedded. The practical importance of the epidural space and its contents for LP lies in the possibility of inadvertently puncturing the venous plexus, or more rarely, one of the small arteries, resulting in a "bloody tap." Striking the roots of a segmental nerve in its sleeve is another mishap that may lead to long lasting paresthesias. In the epidural space the roots surrounded by their meningeal sleeve are relatively fixed and cannot as easily evade the needle as in the subarachnoid space.

In passing, it may be mentioned that the epidural space is not infrequently utilized as the site of epidural (peridural) anesthesia of the segmental nerves. This procedure should not be confused with intrathecal (spinal) anesthesia in which the anesthetizing fluid is injected into the subarachnoid space. In caudal anesthesia, the needle is inserted through the sacral hiatus into the distal part of the sacral canal without penetrating the dural sac, which ends at the second sacral vertebra. It is a useful method of obtaining analgesia in obstetrics.

Subdural and subarachnoid spaces

The next step in LP after the ligamentum flavum has been penetrated and the epidural space passed, is the piercing of the dura/arachnoid, which again may be perceived as a "snap." The needle now is in the subarachnoid space, and under normal conditions spinal fluid will appear at the hub of the needle (Figs. 1 and 2). The pressure of the spinal fluid should be determined and its clearness, color, cell and protein count investigated. Fluid for bacterial cultures also should be collected. Is there a subdural space between dura and arachnoid? There is a capillary interval containing a minimal amount of fluid for lubrication of the contiguous aspects of the two membranes.

Lateral approach in LP

In older people or people with metabolic disease, the supraspinal ligament may be ossified or calcified and perforation by the puncture needle may become difficult. Such a calcified ligament may also deflect the needle from its intended course so that it strikes the bony laminae above or below the puncture site. In this case a slightly lateral approach to one side of the midline may be chosen (Fig. 2). Since the lower lamina rises upward from the midline, the needle is directed slightly cranially to miss the lamina of the lower vertebra and slightly medially to compensate for the lateral point of entrance. In this approach the needle passes through skin, a variable amount of superficial fascia and fat, the dense posterior layer of the thoracolumbar fascia, and the erector spinae muscles. The needle now has to penetrate only the ligamentum flavum (since the supra- and interspinal ligaments have been bypassed), the epidural space, and the dura/arachnoid before spinal fluid escapes.

Side effects and complications

Several of the side effects have already been mentioned, such as a bloody tap due to puncture of the epidural venous plexus, and acute root pain or longer-lasting neuralgia of a spinal nerve caused by contact with or injury by the needle.

A most serious and often fatal complication is prolapse of the temporal lobe or cerebellum with compression of the vital centers of the brain stem in patients with increased intracranial pressure. This also has been discussed previously. If the needle passes through an infected area or a faulty, nonsterile tech-

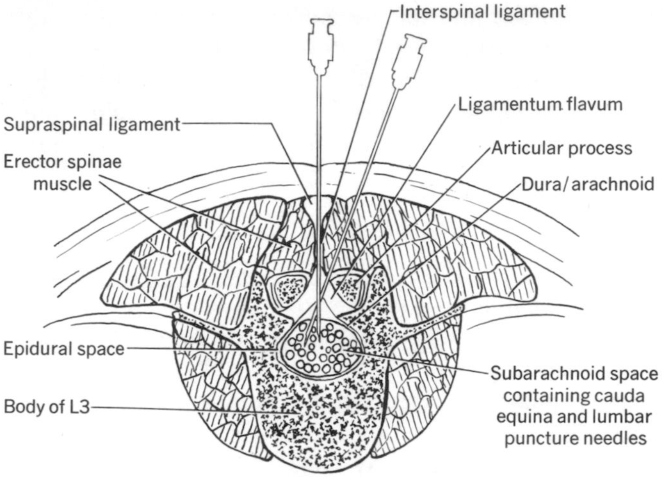

Figure 2—Horizontal section through the body of L3. Notice two puncture needles in the subarachnoid space. The medial one is in the midline corresponding to the position in Figure 1. The lateral exemplifies the lateral approach which avoids the occasionally calcified supraspinal ligament. Notice the lateral needle piercing the intrinsic musculature of the back and only one ligament, the ligamentum flavum.

nique is employed, septic meningitis may result. Other incidents are puncture of the posterior longitudinal ligament and the anulus fibrosus, resulting in prolapse of the nucleus pulposus of the intervertebral disk. One author compiled fifty-seven cases of this type of injury from the literature and his own experience. Surprisingly, the literature also reports the presence of bone-marrow cells in the spinal fluid due to penetration of the vertebral body by the puncture needle.

Post-puncture headache

However, the most frequent side effect is postpuncture headache. This is slow in starting, taking two to three days to reach its peak. The pain is caused by leakage of CSF at the site of puncture of the dura, resulting in decreased hydrostatic pressure in the subarachnoid space. This leads to slight dislodgement of the brain and traction on pain-sensitive blood vessels and intracranial dura. The brain itself does not perceive pain. The headache is increased in the erect position and temporarily relieved by a second LP with injection of saline solution. Horizontal position, with the patient's head flat and unsupported by pillows, alleviates it. The headache generally lasts only a few days. It is obvious that small gauge puncture needles and avoidance of multiple punctures will alleviate or prevent postpuncture headache.

12 Psoas Abscess

A 20-year-old male Indian is transferred to the University Hospital from a sanatorium for tuberculous patients, where he has been for a year with a diagnosis of pulmonary tuberculosis. Several years earlier his grandmother died of tuberculosis of the lung. For the preceding six months he has complained of backache, which has become more severe during the last few weeks. He also has lost weight and suffers from cough and night sweats.

EXAMINATION

On physical examination the patient appears poorly nourished, and shows evidence of tuberculous involvement of the upper right pulmonary lobe, which is confirmed by X-ray examination. There is marked pain in the area of the lower thoracic and upper lumbar spinal column, and tenderness over the spinous processes of the last thoracic and first lumbar vertebrae. The right hip is flexed and externally rotated. Forceful extension of the right thigh is painful and is resisted by the patient. There is present a reducible, painless, fist-sized swelling in the femoral triangle. There also is some fullness in the right iliac fossa. Roentgen examination of the spinal column shows an area of destruction on the right side of the anterior portions of the twelfth thoracic and first lumbar vertebrae, with narrowing of the intervertebral disk space between these two vertebrae. There is a slight left and posteriorly convex angulation of the spinal column corresponding to the area of destruction. In the anteroposterior view there is noted a right-sided bulging of the lateral contour of the psoas shadow.

DIAGNOSIS

Pulmonary tuberculosis, moderately advanced in the right upper lobe. Tuberculosis of the twelfth thoracic intervertebral disk with involvement of the adjacent vertebrae. Right-sided psoas abscess becoming superficial in the femoral triangle.

THERAPY AND FURTHER COURSE

During the next eight weeks the patient is put on specific chemotherapy, including antibiotics for his lung and bone tuberculosis. A nutritious diet and bed rest on a hard mattress are also prescribed. Under this treatment the patient improves, he gains some weight, and his cough subsides.

Under general anesthesia an operation is performed. The retroperitoneal area is entered through a large oblique incision parallel to and one fingerbreadth above the iliac crest. The three anterolateral muscles of the abdominal wall and the transversalis fascia are divided without opening the peritoneal cavity or entering the kidney bed. The fascial covering of the psoas is brought into view by blunt dissection and the psoas fascia divided in order to expose the tuberculous abscess within the psoas compartment. Following the pathway of the abscess on its way downward beneath the inguinal ligament, the latter is also divided. A second incision is made over the femoral triangle to expose the extension of the psoas abscess to the area of the lesser trochanter. The whole extent of the fascial sac, with the abscess and surrounding scar tissue, is excised. The area of destruction in the twelfth thoracic disk and the adjacent two vertebrae is now approached and curetted (scraped), and the infected material and debris are cleaned out. During this procedure care is taken not to injure the right ureter. With this in mind, a catheter has been inserted into it previously. The inferior vena cava, the testicular vessels, and the exposed branches of the lumbar plexus are also identified and protected. Antibiotic solution is injected into the large wound, and soft rubber drains are placed into the upper and lower margins of the incision. The divided transversalis fascia and the three abdominal muscles, the subcutaneous tissue, and skin are sutured. The patient is put in a body cast and strict bed rest is prescribed. Chemotherapy, including antibiotics, is continued for another eight months. Four months after the excisional surgery just described, a fusion operation is done which unites the spinous processes and laminae of the diseased vertebrae with a bone graft taken from the tibia of the patient, the purpose of this surgery being permanent immobilization of the involved vertebrae. The cast and bed rest are continued for another six months after the fusion operation. The patient is then gradually allowed to get up and walk, using a brace.

Examinations, one year and two years after operation, show the patient fully active and employed. He has gained twenty-five pounds, his general status is improved, and his tuberculosis in lung and spinal column seems arrested.

DISCUSSION

We are dealing here with a tuberculous infection of a circumscribed area of the spinal column that has led secondarily to an involvement of the posteromedial portions of the abdominal wall, posterior to the peritoneal cavity, and posteromedial to the kidney and its fascia.

Psoas muscle, fascia and compartment

The affected area can be designated as the psoas compartment since it comprises the psoas major muscle and its fascia and extends downward to the insertion of the iliopsoas muscle (Figs. 1 and 2). Where is the psoas major located? Where does it arise and insert? What is its nerve supply and main action?

The psoas major is a thick fleshy muscle (the fillet of the butcher) that lies in a trough between the bodies and trans-

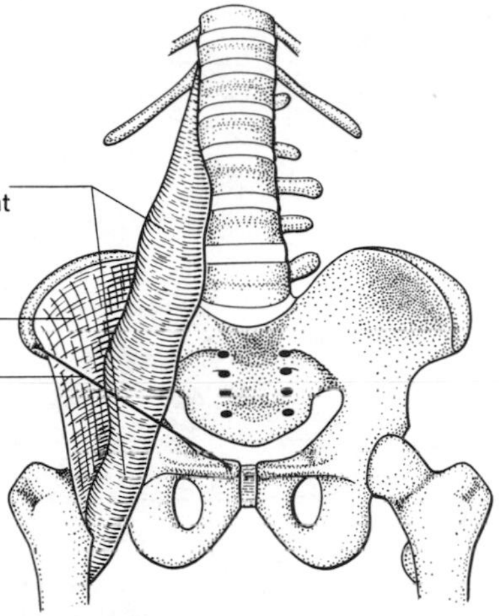

Figure 1—A psoas abscess that originated in the spinal column and broke into the psoas compartment. Notice the bulging of this compartment and the extent of the abscess which reaches under the inguinal ligament into the femoral triangle in front of the trochanter minor.

verse processes of the lumbar vertebrae. The muscle has a continuous origin from the twelfth thoracic to the upper half of the fifth lumbar vertebra, where it arises from the lateral surface of the vertebral bodies, the transverse processes, and the intervening intervertebral disks. It also takes origin from four fibrous arches which bridge the waist of the vertebral bodies and transmit the four lumbar arteries and veins and rami communicantes to the lumbar nerves. The muscle courses downward, forward, and laterally, and passes into the thigh beneath the inguinal ligament just lateral to the iliopectineal eminence (identify the latter on the skeleton). It fuses with the tendon of the iliacus and inserts into the anterior surface of the lesser trochanter of the femur. The muscle is innervated by direct branches of the lumbar plexus. It is the most powerful flexor of the thigh, and when acting from its insertion, it flexes the lumbar spinal column and bends it toward the same side.

What is meant by the term psoas fascia? What is the extent of this fascia and its clinical importance? The anterior surface

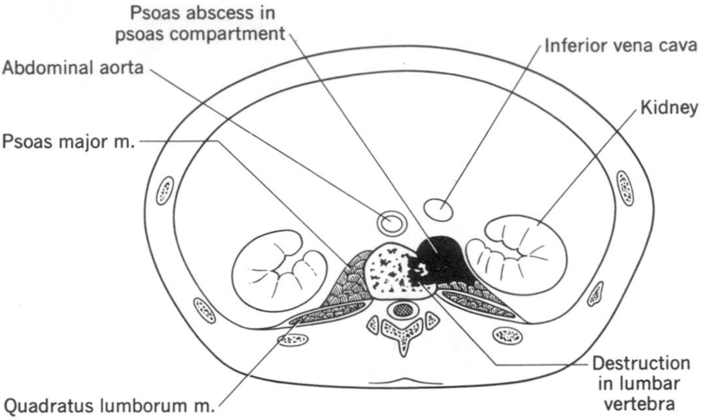

Figure 2—A cross-section at the level of the first lumbar vertebra in the same case. Notice the destruction of the right side of the vertebra with rupture into the psoas compartment. Notice how the psoas abscess causes a bulging of the psoas fascia.

of the psoas major is invested by a well-defined, thin, but fairly strong fascia, the psoas fascia or sheath. Through the fascia of the quadratus lumborum above and the fascia of the iliacus muscle below, the psoas fascia is continuous with the transversalis fascia, which forms the inner lining of the abdominal wall. A cranial thickening of the psoas fascia, which extends from the body of the second lumbar vertebra medially to the transverse process of the first lumbar vertebra laterally, forms the medial lumbocostal arch from which part of the diaphragm arises. This arch, together with the cranial-most portion of the psoas muscle, forms a funnel-shaped orifice that opens cranially into the posterior mediastinum and caudally into the psoas compartment underneath the psoas fascia. It serves as a portal of entrance for pus originating from diseased thoracic vertebrae. Under the influence of a bacterial infection, which is most often tuberculous, the fascia becomes inflamed and thickens, and thus retains the accumulated pus under the clinical picture of a psoas abscess. Gradually destroying the psoas muscle itself and following gravity, the abscess descends within the psoas compartment and frequently becomes superficial in the femoral triangle in front of the insertion of the psoas into the lesser trochanter beneath the fascia lata (Figs. 1 and 2). The medial boundary of the psoas compartment in the abdomen corresponds to the attachment of the psoas muscle and fascia to the spinal column. In the greater pelvis the psoas fascia is continuous anterolaterally with the denser iliac fascia, which attaches to the crest of the ilium. Medially the fascia is inserted here into the pelvic brim or terminal line. Thus, an osseofascial compartment is formed which opens beneath the inguinal ligament into the femoral triangle but is separated from the lesser pelvis by the attachment of the iliopsoas fascia to the pelvic brim.

Anatomy of a typical psoas abscess

How do you visualize the pathological pathway of the disease in our case? As the tuberculous infection leads to destruction of the twelfth thoracic intervertebral disk and the adjacent vertebrae, these structures are no longer able to sustain the weight of the overlying column and partially collapse at the site of the disease. This explains the roentgenographic appearance of narrowing of the disk and partial destruction of the adjacent vertebrae, with distortion of the axis of the spinal column at this point. The partial collapse of the vertebrae squeezes bony debris and pus into the region of least resistance, that is, into the adjacent psoas compartment.

Why does the abscess of the spine not invade the spinal canal posteriorly or the region immediately anterior to the spinal column? The anterior and posterior longitudinal ligaments offer resistance to the spread of the tuberculous process.

Do we have radiographic findings in our case indicating that the tuberculous abscess has invaded the psoas compartment? The lateral margin of the psoas in the normal is demonstrable on the roentgenogram as a straight (non-curving) and laterally descending line that extends from the level of the first lumbar vertebra to the pelvis. In our case, the right psoas margin is characterized by a curving contour corresponding to the bulge of the psoas abscess.

How do you explain the flexed and laterally rotated position of the thigh, a position which the patient naturally assumes and tries to maintain by external support? This position relaxes the muscle and is an attempt to relieve the muscular tension and prevent pressure on the lumbar nerves in the psoas compartment.

Lumbar plexus

What are the nerves in the psoas compartment? They are branches of the lumbar plexus which are also exposed to injury during surgery for psoas abscess. Which is the most important nerve and what is its location in relation to the psoas muscle? The femoral nerve is the principal structure that may be paralyzed in this disease or may be injured during surgery. It lies in the groove between psoas major and iliacus and has to be closely guarded during surgical exposure. Other branches of the lumbar plexus liable to be exposed in radical surgery for psoas abscess are the iliohypogastric and ilioinguinal nerves, which pass under the medial lumbocostal arch, and the lateral femoral cutaneous nerve. These three nerves likewise lie lateral to the psoas major muscle. A fifth nerve, the genitofemoral nerve, pierces the anterior surface of the psoas muscle as well as its fascia and may be damaged by disease or surgery, but this is not of serious consequence. The last, but important nerve of the lumbar plexus, the obturator nerve, lies outside the field of surgery along the medial border of the psoas muscle.

Other pathways of psoas abscess

Can you conceive of any other pathway that a psoas abscess may follow besides the one that has been described? In general it can be stated that the pus collections follow the lines of least resistance. Their position and extent, therefore, are greatly affected by fascial planes and fascial attachments. An example of the latter is the rarity with which a psoas abscess breaks into the lesser pelvis. The firm attachment of the iliopsoas fascia to the pelvic brim precludes the entrance of the abscess into the lesser pelvis. The resistance of the peritoneum makes perforation into the peritoneal cavity and involvement of the intraperitoneal organs an exceptional event.

On the other hand, body position of the patient, such as the upright posture or lateral decubitus (lying on one side) will facilitate extension of the abscess in the corresponding direction. Thus it may spread laterally under the fascia of the quadratus lumborum and come to the surface in the lumbar triangle, leading to an outpouching of the thin floor of this triangle. What muscle forms the floor and what structures form the boundaries of this triangle? The internal abdominal oblique muscle forms the floor, and the latissimus dorsi, the external oblique, and the crest of the ilium form the boundaries of this triangle. A psoas abscess may also extend laterally under the iliacus fascia to appear just medial to the anterior superior iliac spine. Following the usual course into the femoral triangle the abscess may not stop there but track along the medial femoral circumflex vessels and present itself along the posterior aspect of the thigh or perforate there. Or the abscess may follow the femoral vessels through the adductor canal and appear in the popliteal fossa.

What are the boundaries, floor, and content of the femoral triangle, which is so important in this case history? It is bounded laterally by the medial border of the sartorius, medially by the medial border of the adductor longus, and cranially by the inguinal ligament. The iliopsoas, pectineus, and adductor longus form its floor, and the fascia lata its roof. Important contents of the triangle are the femoral nerve and femoral vessels, which have to be protected in surgery draining a psoas abscess. After the femoral vessels leave the apex of the femoral triangle, they enter the adductor canal, which extends from the apex of the femoral triangle to the opening in the adductor magnus by which the femoral vessels appear in the popliteal fossa.

What are the boundaries of the adductor canal? The vastus

medialis bounds it anterolaterally, the adductor longus and magnus posteromedially, while the fascial bridge uniting these boundaries forms the roof of the canal, covered by the sartorius. This then is the pathway that an occasional psoas abscess takes on its way to the popliteal fossa. In rare cases the vertebral abscess may break through the posterior longitudinal ligament into the spinal canal, with consequent involvement of the spinal cord. It may also penetrate through the anterior longitudinal ligament in front of the spinal column and following gravity track down with the aorta and its terminal branches to reach the gluteal region, either cranial or caudal to the piriformis muscle. It arrives there with the terminal branches of the internal iliac artery, that is, the superior or inferior gluteal arteries.

One final pathway should be mentioned since it has important anatomical and clinical implications: that is, the involvement of the iliopectineal bursa by a psoas abscess. This bursa is one of the largest and most important in the human body. Where is it located? It lies in front of the capsule of the hip joint where the iliopsoas tendon passes adjacent to the iliopectineal eminence. Does this bursa communicate with the hip joint? In 10 to 15 per cent, it opens into the joint. If a psoas abscess breaks into the bursa, it may involve the hip joint and lead to the serious complication of tuberculosis of the hip joint.

This case serves as an instructive example of the clinically well-known fact that the spread of abscesses frequently is determined by fascial attachments and that knowledge of fascial anatomy allows us to predict the various pathways that abscesses may take. This also holds true for the fascial compartments in the neck where the anatomy of the different layers of cervical fascia affects the direction of the spread of infections, including the entrance of pus into the mediastinum.

Thoracic Viscera

13 Segmental Abscess of Lung

A farm boy, age 18, comes to the hospital because of cough and foul expectoration. He complains of great weakness and continual cough with expectoration of a dark yellow, foul-smelling mucous substance, and pain along the right upper chest wall, particularly under the right scapula. His trouble began two days after a tonsillectomy, under ether anesthesia, five weeks earlier. It started as a sharp pain in the chest, which was made worse by deep inspiration. The cough did not begin until about two weeks after the first attack of pain. About the time he began to cough, he felt that he had a fever.

EXAMINATION

On examination his temperature is 105° and he has a leukocytosis. Radiographic examination in front and side views shows an abscess cavity with fluid in the right posterior upper area of the chest (see Fig. 1). Visibility of the interlobar fissures on profile X-ray view makes it possible to locate the abscess in the posterior segment of the upper lobe.

DIAGNOSIS

Segmental abscess of the lung.

The history of this case, greatly modified, is taken from A. E. Hertzler: Clinical Surgery by Case Histories, St. Louis, C. V. Mosby Company, 1921, vol. 1, p. 280.

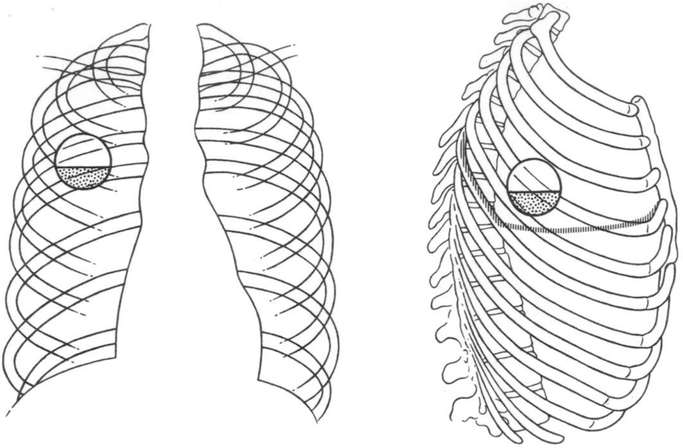

Figure 1—Abscess cavity with fluid level in the posterior segment of the right upper lobe on front and side view.

THERAPY AND FURTHER COURSE

The abscess completely cleared up under vigorous antibiotic therapy. Three months later the healing was complete and the patient was free from any symptoms.

DISCUSSION

Tonsillectomy not infrequently leads to inhalation of infected material from the throat during general anesthesia, resulting in lung abscess.

Anatomy of segmental abscess

In the supine position of the body during and after surgery the posterior segments of the lungs are particularly endangered; indeed the posterior segment of the upper lobe is the most common site of pulmonary abscess. What posterior segments of the lower lobe may also be involved? The apical and posterior basal segments of the lower lobe could readily be infected in the supine position of the body. If surgery should become necessary, from what thoracic region would you enter the diseased segment, keeping in mind that the involved segment should be attacked from its pleural aspect, and without proceeding through uninvolved segments? The posterior approach would best fulfill these requirements. It is important to realize that, as in this case, the upper lobe may reach caudally on the posterior chest wall as far down as the sixth rib. Is that in keeping with your textbook diagrams? Textbook figures, based on the cadaveric position of the lungs in maximal expiration, generally show the oblique fissures being projected on the posterior thoracic wall at the level of the fourth rib or fourth interspace.

Pleural pain

Since the lung and visceral pleura themselves are insensitive to pain, how do you explain the severe pain of the patient? In contrast to the visceral pleura, the parietal pleura, particularly in its costal portion, is very sensitive to pain which may be intensified by spasms in the overlying muscles of the chest wall. What nerves transmit this pain from the parietal pleura? The costal and peripheral parts of the diaphragmatic pleura are supplied with sensory fibers from the intercostal and subcostal nerves. The central portion of the diaphragmatic pleura and the mediastinal pleura receive their sensory supply from the phrenic nerve. This pain is often referred to neck and shoulder.

14 Middle Lobe Syndrome

A 32-year-old housewife comes to the chest clinic with a history of chronic cough and blood-tinged sputum. The symptoms began eight months earlier when she had an acute flu-like respiratory infection with fever and expectoration. Since that time she has suffered from bouts of fever which occur every two to three weeks. These episodes are accompanied by right-sided chest pain and production of a large amount of purulent and frequently blood-tinged sputum. She has lost eighteen pounds of weight. She feels very tired and is hardly able to do her housework. The patient is admitted to the hospital for diagnosis.

EXAMINATION

On examination her chest findings are minimal. On auscultation of the chest there are found some abnormal breath sounds over the lower anterior portion of the right chest. The temperature is 98.8°. The sputum is negative for tubercle bacilli.

Roentgen films of the chest in front and profile views reveal infiltration and partial collapse of the right middle lobe (Fig. 1). Examination of the right bronchus with a bronchoscope shows narrowing and inflammation of the mucosa of the middle lobe bronchus, from which exudes a purulent secretion. Roentgenographic visualization of the right bronchial tree with injection of a radio-opaque iodized oil (bronchography) shows partial obliteration of the right middle lobe bronchus which prevents distinct filling of its branches.

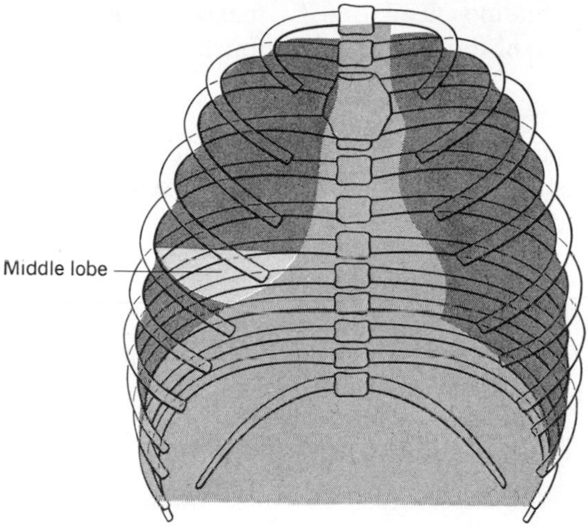

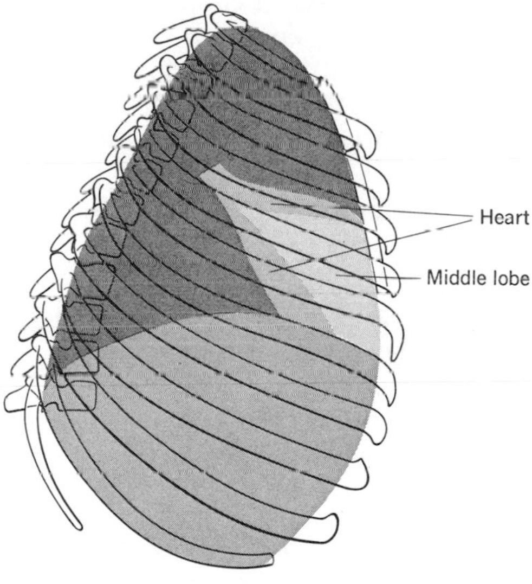

Figure 1 shows the partially atelectatic and infiltrated middle lobe as it appears on posteroanterior and lateral roentgenograms.

These findings lead one to make a tentative diagnosis of obstruction of the middle lobe bronchus.

DIAGNOSIS

We are dealing here with an interesting clinical and pathological entity that has become known recently as the "middle lobe syndrome."

THERAPY AND FURTHER COURSE

After the diagnostic work-up is completed, the patient is admitted to the thoracic surgical service for operation. Righsided thoracotomy is performed. The thorax is opened through the right fifth intercostal space with the patient in semi-lateral position. The right middle lobe is found to be partially collapsed and consolidated. There are numerous enlarged lymph nodes surrounding the middle lobe bronchus. The middle lobe is resected, after its bronchus and artery and the veins draining it have been ligated. Study of the excised lobe reveals that the lobe is the site of chronic infection with many inflammatory changes. The lobe also shows numerous dilated bronchi (bronchiectasis).

The postoperative course is uneventful and the patient is discharged ten days after operation. Repeated examinations at three-month intervals show that the patient is relieved of all her symptoms and has regained her previous weight.

DISCUSSION

The sequence of events generally starts with a bacterial infection of the lung, which then spreads along lymphatic channels to regional lymph nodes at the root of the lung. These nodes become inflamed and enlarged. Later on the nodes, increased in size, may harden or even become calcified and compress the middle lobe bronchus.

Lymphatic channels

What is the chain of lymph nodes that drains the lung, bronchi, and visceral pleura? A few lymph nodes, called pulmonary nodes, are located within the substance of the lung along the larger bronchi near the hilus. They drain into bronchopulmonary nodes at the hilus of the lung. Their lymph is received by the superior and inferior tracheobronchial nodes, with the former lying in the angle between trachea and main bronchi and the latter within the bifurcation of the trachea. In turn their efferent vessels transport lymph into a group of nodes distributed along each side of the trachea, called tracheal nodes (Fig. 2). Efferent lymph vessels of the tracheal nodes and direct lymph channels from the tracheobronchial nodes join lymphatics from nodes that drain mediastinal organs to form the right and left bronchomediastinal trunks. These commonly open into the venous angle formed by the internal jugular and subclavian veins. Less frequently the right trunk may drain into the right lymphatic and the left into the thoracic duct.

Obstruction of the middle lobe bronchus

The compression of a lobar bronchus by enlarged lymph nodes, leading to bronchostenosis, may occur at the site of any lobar bronchus but is most common at the middle lobe bronchus. Are there any features in the anatomy of the middle lobe bronchus that make it particularly susceptible to stenosis and compression by enlarged lymph nodes? The answer is in the affirmative. The stem of the middle lobe bronchus descends forward and downward before it divides, and during this course it is encircled by a group of lymph nodes which, when enlarged, may reach cherry size (Fig. 2). Other lobar bronchi do not enter into such close relationship with nodes and are therefore not as liable to be compressed.

Do these nodes that surround the middle lobe bronchus drain the middle lobe exclusively? Lymphatic drainage does not strictly follow a lobar pattern. Each lung can be subdivided into three zones of lymphatic drainage which do not coincide with the lobar boundaries. Thus the lymph nodes around the middle lobe bronchus receive lymph not only from the middle lobe but also from adjacent portions of the lower lobe. It is therefore conceivable that a primary infec-

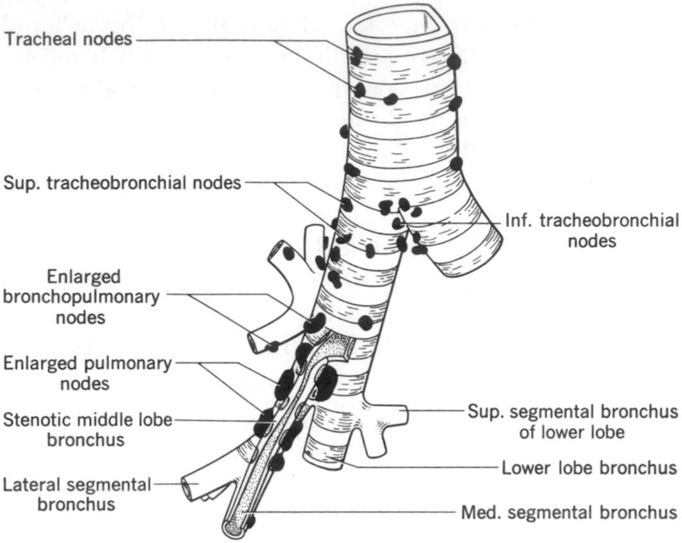

Figure 2 shows the opened middle lobe bronchus partially obstructed by enlarged lymph nodes and the chains of lymph nodes associated with trachea and bronchi. Tracheobronchial tree is rotated to the right.

tion of the lower lobe may lead to enlargement of lymph nodes that compress and obstruct the middle lobe bronchus with the typical consequences of chronic stenosis of this bronchus.

Partial occlusion of the middle lobe bronchus may allow air to enter but prevent it from leaving, since inspiratory forces are stronger. This results in an overdistention of the air spaces in the middle lobe (emphysema). On the other hand, if the obstruction is complete the air is absorbed by the capillaries of the lung and the lumen collapses (atelectasis). If infection enters a lobe that is supplied by a partially obstructed bronchus a vicious circle is set up. This consists of pulmonary infection being followed by further lymph node enlargement with increase in the bronchostenosis, which prevents drainage of the accumulated pus from the involved lobe. Destructive changes in the lung parenchyma follow, leading to chronic suppuration and tissue breakdown. This is accompanied by dilatation of the bronchi whose walls are damaged by the infection (bronchiectasis). Lung abscesses and pleurisy may also be part of the clinical picture. Our case shows many of the signs mentioned, particularly infection of the middle lobe parenchyma, bronchiectasis, and pleurisy. The latter could be predicted from the preoperatively present pleural pain, the former from the fever, malaise, weight loss, and the large amount of purulent and sometimes bloody sputum expectorated from the middle lobe.

Frequently, particularly in children, the enlargement of the lymph nodes compressing the middle lobe bronchus may be due to tuberculosis, which has a predilection for lymphatic spread.

Applied anatomy of the middle lobe and its bronchi

Is the direction of the middle lobe bronchus conducive to easy drainage from the infected lobe? The middle lobe bronchus originates from the main bronchus at a rather acute angle and takes a distinctly caudal direction, which certainly makes drainage more difficult. Some observers call attention to the length and pliability of the bronchus, which facilitates compression by encircling nodes. The factors listed are responsible for the clinical and pathological entity that is represented by our case and with which we have recently become familiar through published case histories. How long is the middle lobe bronchus? Name the segmental bronchi into which it divides. The middle lobe bronchus has an average length of about 1.8 cm., after which course it divides into its two segmental branches, the medial and lateral bronchus. The medial bronchus runs downward and forward, the lateral bronchus downward, forward, and laterally. The course of these segmental bronchi is of importance, as is the shape of the segments supplied by them, since these segments may be the site of isolated collapse due to compression of the segmental bronchi by enlarged lymph nodes. The identification of the involved segments can be made from anteroposterior and lateral roentgenograms. But it may be helpful to visualize these segments as being located anteromedially and posterolaterally, realizing that the terms "anterior" and "posterior" apply only to their relation to each other within the lobe. Both segments are, of course, located in front of the oblique fissure, as is the whole middle lobe. Do both segments come in contact with the diaphragm, with only pleura intervening, or are they separated from the diaphragm by the basal segments of the lower lobe? Unless they are retracted by collapse or by pleural adhesions, both segments are directly related to the diaphragm.

How do you approach the medial and lateral segments surgically? Would you ever go through the posterior chest wall in your approach to them? The medial segment is best approached from the front just below the level of the horizontal fissure, which approximately coincides with the fourth costal cartilage. The lateral segment is attacked surgically from the axillary region. Here it lies in front of the lower part of the oblique fissure, whose level roughly coincides with the course of the sixth rib.

What segmental bronchus of the lower lobe has its origin almost directly opposite the origin of the middle lobe bronchus, so that infected material from the diseased segment may readily enter the middle lobe bronchus and lead to secondary involvement of this lobe? The superior bronchus of the lower lobe arises opposite the middle lobe bronchus. Pus and infected sputum from the superior (apical) segment of the lower lobe are particularly apt to enter the middle lobe bronchus if the patient with an apical abscess of the lower lobe is placed in the prone position (chest down) for purposes of drainage of this abscess.

Keeping in mind that the middle lobe is bounded by the horizontal fissure cranially and the oblique fissure posterolaterally, what would be the shape of an infected lobe on posteroanterior and lateral roentgenograms? The posteroanterior roentgenogram shows a dense quadrilateral shadow with a sharp, upper horizontal boundary corresponding to the horizontal fissure. The shadow fades out caudolaterally since it is overlapped here by normal air-containing lung. The lateral roentgenogram is more revealing and displays a triangular shadow whose apex points posteriorly and whose superior and posterolateral boundaries are formed by the horizontal and oblique fissures bordering on normal air-containing lung tissue of the upper and lower lobes (Fig. 1).

15 Lung Cancer with Metastasis

A 56-year-old bookkeeper is referred to the hospital by his family physician. His symptoms consist of persistent cough producing blood-tinged sputum and discomfort in the left chest. He also complains of respiratory wheezing and some shortness of breath. The symptoms started about six months ago and have gradually worsened. His çough keeps him awake at night. His appetite is greatly diminished and he has lost twenty pounds.

EXAMINATION

Physical examination of this rather emaciated and weak-appearing patient showed dullness on percussion over the lower posterior portions of the left lung and absence of breath sounds over the same area on auscultation.

Complete roentgen study of his chest revealed collapse of the left lower lobe. There was widening of the upper right mediastinum which was bounded toward the lung by a lobulated margin. It was assumed that this widening was caused by a cluster of enlarged tracheal lymph nodes. Bronchography with radiopaque oil revealed an intraluminal obstruction of the left lower lobe bronchus. Bronchoscopy visualized an obstructive tumor in the left lower lobe bronchus (Fig. 1) and afforded an opportunity for removal of a biopsy specimen. The biopsy revealed a squamous cell carcinoma.

DIAGNOSIS

Bronchogenic carcinoma in the left lower bronchus with bronchial obstruction and collapse of the left lower lobe.

FURTHER COURSE AND THERAPY

During the next two weeks the patient developed a spiking fever which was probably caused by a superimposed infection in the collapsed lobe. His sputum increased in amount and he was put on antibiotics. In view of the probable cancerous involvement of the mediastinal lymph nodes on the contralateral side, radical surgery, consisting of removal of the left lung and all accessible lymph nodes, did not seem to offer a good chance for cure. However, biopsy of the scalene (supraclavicular) nodes on both sides was undertaken in order to assess the prognosis for this patient by determining the presence or absence of cancerous invasion of these nodes. They were found to be involved on both sides. Thus, radical resection of the left lung was ruled out and radiation treatment was given. Under this treatment the patient improved temporarily. Inquiry, however, revealed that he died six months later at another hospital. At autopsy, a large tumor was found which occluded the left lower lobe bronchus (Fig. 1). It penetrated the bronchial wall and invaded the surrounding lung parenchyma. The rest of the lobe was collapsed and showed signs of infection and scarring. Numerous cancerous lymph nodes were found in both hilar regions and on both sides of the trachea. There also was metastatic involvement of brain and adrenals.

DISCUSSION

The Anatomy and Results of Surgical Treatment of Bronchogenic Cancer

We are dealing here with a bronchogenic cancer, which in men who smoke heavily is the most common cancer. Only in a third of the patients with lung cancer is surgical treatment possible and with it the chance of a cure. In the other two-

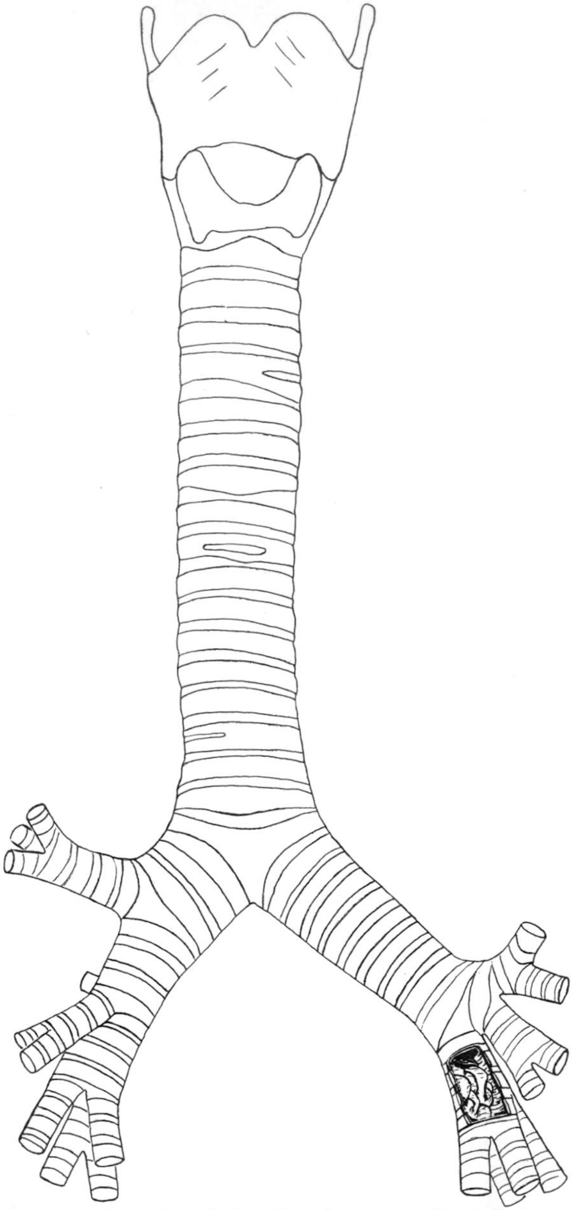

Figure 1 demonstrates the obstructive tumor in the left lower lobe bronchus.

thirds treatment, including radiation therapy, can only be palliative, designed to relieve suffering and make death easier. In the operable patients, removal of a whole lung (pneumonectomy) rather than of only a lobe (lobectomy) is the rule. By its nature, pneumonectomy includes ligation and subsequent division of the pulmonary artery, two pulmonary veins, and a main bronchus. In addition, all accessible regional lymph nodes are excised. A more radical version of this operation includes block dissection in one piece of the bifurcation nodes, the tracheal nodes on both sides, and as many mediastinal nodes of the opposite side as possible. Lobectomy, on the other hand, is resorted to as a curative procedure for tumors of limited extent without or with minimal involvement of the regional nodes or, in more advanced cases, as a palliative measure in patients with poor respiratory or cardiac reserve. The main danger of both operations is leakage of the bronchial stump, i.e. a bronchopleural fistula and infection of the pleural cavity. The five-year survival rate of all patients with pulmonary cancer, including inoperable cases, is 6 to 8 per cent. However, 21 to 30 per cent of the patients, who were operated, were alive after five years.

The Pulmonary Lymphatic System in Cancer Spread

The pulmonary lymphatic system is the most important channel of spread of lung cancer. It has been said that the surgery of malignant disease is not so much the surgery of the involved organs, but more so of the lymphatic system draining these organs. This statement applies particularly well to cancer of the lung, where the chance for cure and survival is essentially dependent on the anatomy of lymphatic cancer spread. Cancerous involvement of the lymph vessels and subsequent dissemination via these channels to the hilar and mediastinal nodes are the most important modes of cancer dispersal (metastasis). Direction of the lymph stream and lymphatic drainage of various regions of the lung are a fixed and inherited characteristic, that does not follow a strict lobar pattern. It allows us to predict with fair accuracy that lymph and abnormal contents of the lymph stream, such as clusters of cancer cells (cancerous emboli), will be carried to specific lymph nodes. However, there are in addition more variable pathways, which, through anastomoses with the typical lymphatic channels, may conduct some of the lymph as well as cancerous emboli into different sets of lymph nodes. For the lung the typical channels are well established and are discussed in the literature (see Case Study 14). They comprise the pulmonary, the bronchopulmonary, the tracheobronchial, and tracheal nodes, listed in the order in which the lymph stream traverses them. The subsidiary or collateral lymphatic pathways, which represent additional channels of lymph drainage of various lung regions, however, are not as well known and are more variable. They are particularly apt to play a role in cancer spread if the typical regional lymph nodes are blocked by cancerous growth. In this case small anatomically preformed or newly formed lymph vessels may open up to bypass the obstructed nodes. Reversal of lymph flow may also occur as well as crossing of the midline by lymph vessels that connect with nodes on the opposite side.

The original breakthrough of cancer of the bronchial mucosa occurs into peribronchial and perivascular lymphatics. From there the spread is generally discontinuous with small masses of cancer cells (emboli) carried with the lymph stream to regional lymph nodes. The typical number of lymph nodes concerned with drainage of the lung is approximately fifty to sixty nodes.

Since the incidence of regional lymph-node involvement (metastasis) at autopsy of lung cancer patients is as high as 95 per cent and in surgical specimen amounts to more than 70 per cent, interest is naturally focused on the path and sequence of intrathoracic lymph node involvement. The following questions and answers may summarize recent findings on this topic.

Question: In cancer of the right upper and middle lobes, which nodes among the *bronchopulmonary chain* are preferentially involved? Answer: The nodes in the angle between right upper and middle lobe bronchi (Fig. 2A).

Question: Which group among the *tracheobronchial nodes* is favored by lymphatic spread from upper or middle lobe cancer? Answer: The inferior tracheobronchial (bifurcation) nodes (Fig. 2B).

Question: Does bypassing of bronchopulmonary nodes and direct spread to tracheobronchial and/or tracheal nodes occur? Answer: It does and is one of the characteristic features of lymphatic spread of pulmonary cancer, regardless of the lobe involved.

Question: Are cancers of the *right upper* lobe liable to spread to bronchopulmonary nodes caudal to the middle lobe bronchus? Answer: This is unlikely.

Question: Which among the bronchopulmonary nodes are commonly involved in cancer of the *left upper* lobe? Answer: Nodes in the angle between the left upper and lower lobe bronchi (Fig. 2C).

Question: Which accessory lymph channel and nodes may often become cancerous in spread from the *left upper* lobe? Answer: An anterior mediastinal channel and subaortic nodes adjacent to the ligamentum arteriosum and the recurrent laryngeal nerve (Fig. 2D).

Question: Which nodes are typically affected in cancer spread from the *right or left lower lobes*? Answer: Bronchopulmonary nodes between middle and lower lobe bronchus on the right (Fig. 2E) and upper and lower lobe bronchus on the left (Fig. 2C), as well as nodes between upper and middle lobe bronchus on the right (Fig. 2A) and above the upper lobe bronchus on the left. Further drainage takes place into superior (Fig. 2F) and inferior tracheobronchial nodes (Fig. 2B), and also to nodes in the pulmonary ligament and posterior mediastinal nodes (not shown in figure).

Question: Is there a difference in the lymphatic drainage of the right and left lower lobes? Answer: Contralateral spread to the right tracheal nodes in cancer of the *left* lower lobe is a common occurrence, while spread to left nodes in right-sided lung cancer seems infrequent.

The latter point is well exemplified by our case of cancer in the left lower lobe bronchus which displays spread to con-

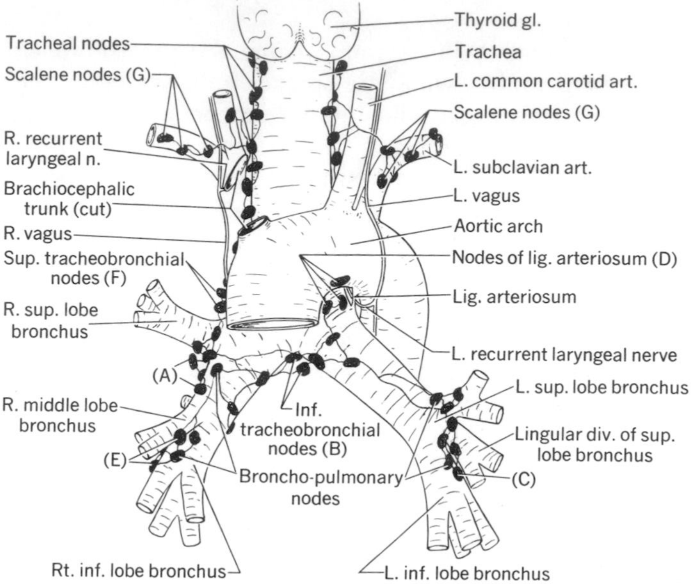

Figure 2 shows the tracheobronchial tree with lymph nodes particularly apt to be involved in the spread of bronchogenic malignancies. For explanation and identification of nodes marked by symbols, see text.

tralateral tracheal lymph nodes on the roentgenogram. The autopsy findings in our patient showed involvement of most of the lymph nodes in the right and left hilar and paratracheal areas. The finding is fairly typical in cases that have terminated fatally.

Scalene node biopsy

Our case history mentions that a scalene node biopsy was done and that the finding of cancer cells in these nodes precluded radical surgery. How is this diagnostic procedure performed? What are its dangers and what is its rationale? Scalene node biopsy for diagnosis of cancer spread from the lung was initiated about twenty-five years ago paralleling the increasing interest in radical pulmonary surgery. The operation, which is done under local anesthesia, consists of removal of deep cervical lymph nodes. After division of skin, platysma, and the appropriate layers of deep cervical fascia, and after medial retraction of the sternocleidomastoid muscle, a pad of fat and embedded lymph vessels and nodes superficial to the scalene muscles are removed *in toto*. The territory involved is bounded by the posterior belly of the omohyoid laterally, the internal jugular vein medially, and the subclavian vein caudally. The operation may require ligation of the external jugular vein and the transverse cervical and suprascapular vessels. Care must be taken not to injure the dome of the parietal pleura, the internal jugular vein, the subclavian vein, the phrenic nerve, the brachial plexus, and the thoracic duct on the left. Identify these structures on atlas pictures and remember that the phrenic nerve lies on the substance of the anterior scalenus muscle deep to the prevertebral fascia. The operation is frequently extended into the upper mediastinum with the aim of removing some of the tracheal nodes as well. Is the scalene node removal always done on the site of the suspected malignancy? Since the lymph from the left lower lobe drains in part at least into the right tracheal nodes and since lymphatic communications across the midline have been demonstrated as subsidiary channels, particularly in the presence of obstruction of the lymph stream, bilateral scalene node biopsy is probably the operation of choice, the more so when the tumor is in the left lower lung region. What is the rationale of the operation and what are the pathways along which these inferior deep cervical (supraclavicular) nodes become involved in cancer of the lung? In answering this question, it must be realized that the trachea is not only a mediastinal, but also a cervical organ and that the tracheal nodes to both sides of this tube extend with the trachea into the neck (Fig. 2G). Collateral channels exist between the cervical tracheal nodes and the nodes in the lower part of the posterior triangle, which are removed in scalene node biopsy (Fig. 2G). How often does this cancerous involvement of the scalene nodes occur? Carcinoma of the lungs yields a positive diagnosis in approximately 40 per cent of all scalene node biopsies. If such metastasis has occurred, the case is regarded as inoperable and opening of the thorax becomes unnecessary. It is worth mentioning that scalene node biopsy is done also in cases of other lung diseases such as sarcoidosis and tumors of the lymphatic system.

Mediastinal complications in lung cancer

Mediastinal lymph node involvement may lead to some noteworthy complications. Mention has been made of spread to a lymph node or nodes in the vicinity of the left recurrent laryngeal nerve. What clinical complications would occur with pressure on this nerve? It would result in hoarseness due to paralysis of the left vocal cord (Fig. 2D). One leaf of the diaphragm may be paralyzed by pressure on the phrenic nerve in case of enlarged and cancerous mediastinal lymph nodes. The latter may also displace the esophagus and cause difficulty in swallowing (dysphagia). This can easily be demonstrated by an X-ray examination, with the patient swallowing an opaque medium. An overexposed chest film may also reveal widening of the angle of bifurcation caused by enlarged inferior tracheobronchial lymph nodes. Finally, the superior vena cava may be obstructed by tumors of the right upper lobe or cancerous invasion of the regional lymph nodes (see Case Study 20).

Vascular spread of lung cancer

In addition to involvement of the lymphatics, erosion of the pulmonary veins in bronchial carcinoma is quite common and of serious consequence, since it leads to dispersal of cancerous emboli through the bloodstream. Describe the pathway along which such emboli from the lung have to travel to reach distant organs throughout the body. After the pulmonary veins have been invaded by cancer, the emboli pass through the left atrium, the left ventricle, and by way of the aorta into the arterial circulation, until they are arrested in the capillary filters of various organs. Such hematogenous metastases are most frequent in the suprarenal glands, the brain, bone, liver, and kidneys.

16 Mediastinal Pleurisy

An eight-month-old infant boy is brought into the out-patient department by his mother with a history of irritability and restlessness for the preceding two months. The mother reports that three months earlier he had a middle ear infection which required lancing of the eardrum and drainage of the middle ear. She also stated that he has been coughing for some time and that his breathing has become noisy and wheezing, particularly at night. He is admitted to the hospital.

EXAMINATION

Examination shows that the infant is well developed, but slightly underweight. His upper respiratory tract is moderately inflamed. He has the physical signs of a bronchitis and a low grade fever.

Radiographic examination of the chest reveals a homogeneous, laterally well defined shadow paralleling the right cardiac margin (Fig. 1). On further fluoroscopic and radiographic study with the patient in various positions, this abnormal radiographic finding is interpreted as an encapsulated effusion, located anteriorly in the lower part of the right pleural cavity between visceral and mediastinal pleura.

DIAGNOSIS

Right-sided anterior-inferior mediastinal pleurisy with exudate.

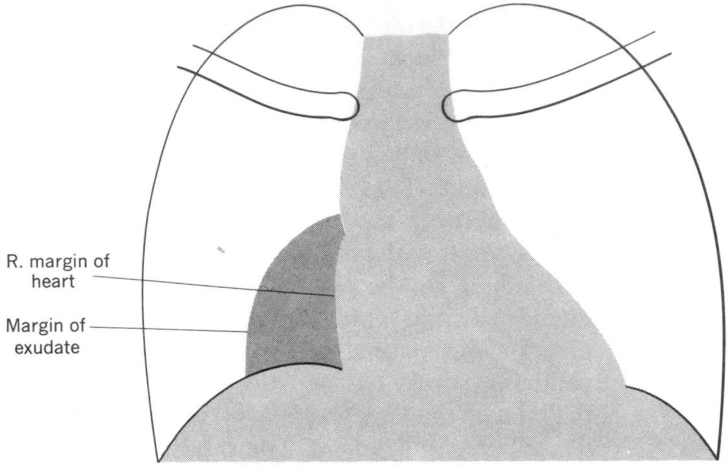

Figure 1—Roentgenogram of chest shows a homogeneous, laterally sharply defined shadow paralleling the right cardiac margin caused by right-sided anterior-inferior mediastinal pleurisy with exudate.

THERAPY AND FURTHER COURSE

The pleural cavity was tapped through the anterior thoracic wall, and 250 cc. of clear fluid were removed. Although no pathogenic organisms could be identified in the fluid, the patient was put on antibiotic and antifebrile medication. During the next two weeks the breathing improved and cough and fever subsided. The subsequent radiographic study showed disappearance of the previously described shadow. The patient was discharged from the hospital.

DISCUSSION

Pleural effusions as a concomitant or result of upper respiratory infections are not an uncommon finding in the infant. What is the content of the normal pleural cavity? The latter is only a potential space containing a thin film of lubricating fluid which facilitates sliding respiratory motion between the two layers of pleura. What are these two layers and at what location are they continuous with each other? Do the pleural cavities of the two sides communicate? What are the subdivisions of the parietal pleura? The visceral pleura which covers each lung is continuous with the parietal pleura as a sleeve around the hilus of the lung and below the hilus as a pleural fold, the pulmonary ligament. The subdivisions of the parietal pleura, which lines the thoracic walls and reaches into the neck above the anterior portion of the first rib, are the cervical, the costal, the diaphragmatic, and the mediastinal pleura. The pleural cavities of the two sides normally do not communicate.

Location of pleural exudates

Exudates as a result of pleural inflammation may collect in the pleural cavity between the previously named parts of the parietal pleura and the visceral pleura. If sufficiently large, the exudate may completely envelop the pleura-ensheathed lung laterally, anteriorly, posteriorly, medially, superiorly, and inferiorly. Frequently, however, with time, more or less broad adhesions between parietal and visceral pleura are formed which localize the exudate in one or more areas. Such encapsulated effusions may, for example, be found between the base of the lung and the diaphragmatic pleura.

Are all pleural exudates fluid collections between parietal and visceral pleura? Interlobar pleurisy results in accumulation of fluid between two layers of visceral pleura in the horizontal and oblique fissures.

Anatomy of mediastinal pleurisy

In infants with respiratory infection, encapsulated fluid collections between the mediastinal and visceral pleura are quite common and are identified as a mediastinal pleurisy. Is this exudate in the mediastinum? The mediastinum is the space between the right and left mediastinal pleurae and is not involved in this affection. The fluid collection is located on either side of the mediastinum.

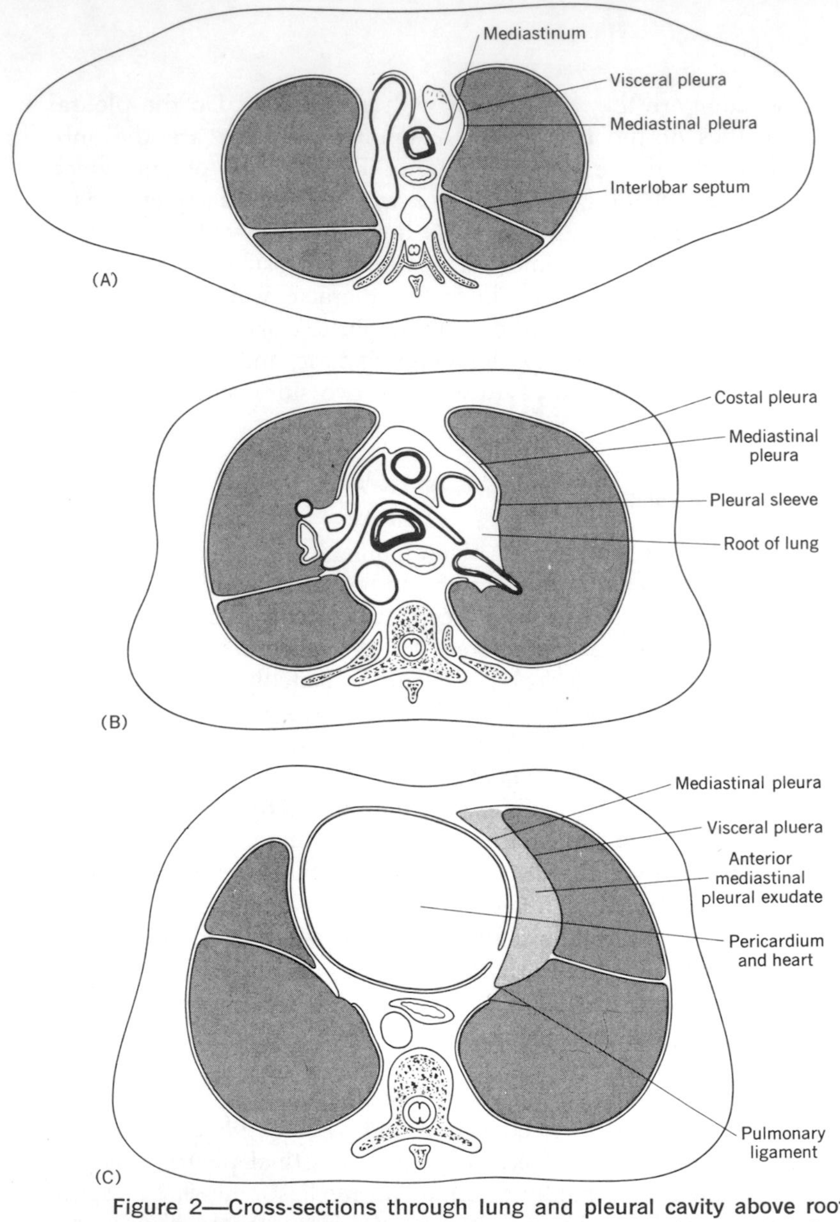

Figure 2—Cross-sections through lung and pleural cavity above root of lung (A), at root of lung (B), and caudal to root of lung at level of pulmonary ligament (C). Note exudate in C in anterior pleuromediastinal space.

For the understanding of the topography of a mediastinal pleurisy it is necessary to visualize the difference in the extent of the mediastinal pleural space at the hilus, and cranial and caudal to it. What is the difference in the cross-sectional arrangement of the pleural space at these three levels (Fig. 2)? Above the hilus of the lung the mediastinal pleural space extends without interruption from the sternum to the spinal column. By contrast, at the hilus and below it the pleural sleeve around the root of the lung and the pulmonary ligament caudal to the root divide the space into anterior and posterior compartments.

Where would effusions between mediastinal and visceral pleura more commonly occupy the whole anteroposterior extent of the pleural space, above or below the root of the lung? While adhesions between the medistinal portion of the parietal and the visceral pleura may confine the extent of the fluid in an anterior or posterior location, for anatomical reasons fluid collections cranial to the hilus frequently are more extensive in a sagittal (anteroposterior) plane than exudates located more caudally. Can you give the boundaries of the fluid collection in the case under discussion (Fig. 2C)? The exudate here is confined by adhesions and normal anatomical boundaries to a part of the right pleural cavity that is bounded anteriorly by sternum and costal cartilages, medially by the lower part of the right mediastinal pleura, caudally by the diaphragmatic pleura, laterally by the medial anterior aspect of the visceral pleura covering the mediastinal surface of the lung, and posteriorly by the pulmonary ligament. The exudate was large enough to displace the right lung laterally to a considerable extent.

Prognosis

In general this type of pleurisy can be regarded as a benign disease whose symptoms gradually disappear under treatment, but which quite often leaves pleural adhesions obliterating the involved part of the pleural cavity.

17 Angina Pectoris

A cook, 59 years old, enters the hospital with a history of attacks of pain that started two years earlier. The pain is located in the left shoulder, radiating from there to the breastbone and to the pit of the stomach. These attacks of pain came at lengthy intervals until the preceding two weeks, when they occurred every day, forcing him to stop work. The pain is not severe and is always relieved by rest. His left arm feels weak, especially after an attack of pain.

EXAMINATION

On physical examination involvement of the joints, muscles, periosteum, and peripheral nerves has to be considered. The shoulder joint shows no objective abnormality and movements are free. Myalgia, a painful condition of the skeletal muscles (the common "charley-horse"), should be thought of, particularly in the older age group whenever unusual physical exercise has preceded the attack of pain. What muscle located in the painful area would be apt to cause a similar distribution of pain? By what motion would you check for non-involvement of this muscle in putting its fibers on the stretch? The fibers of the pectoralis major would be stretched in abduction and lateral rotation of the arm. Absence of pain

Based upon actual case taken from R. C. Cabot's splendid collection of medical case histories in his two-volume work on Differential Diagnosis, third edition, W. B. Saunders Company, Philadelphia, 1915, volume 1, case 176.

in the performance of these motions would rule out inflammation of this muscle.

An inflammatory lesion in the richly innervated periosteum over the ribs can be excluded by the absence of swelling, tenderness and heat. Neuralgia of the intercostal nerves can be ruled out by the absence of pressure pain along the course of the intercostal nerves. How would you check by physical examination for such cause of pain, keeping in mind the course of the intercostal nerves in the area involved? In case of neuralgia of one or more intercostal nerves there would be localized tenderness on pressure along the costal groove and inferior margin of the corresponding ribs.

Further examination shows the heart slightly enlarged, but otherwise negative. Palpation reveals radial and brachial arteries markedly thickened and tortuous.

With reference to the patient's complaint we note that the pain comes in attacks which are relieved by rest, and that it has very wide radiation.

DIAGNOSIS

Pain of the type described in a man of fifty-nine suggests angina pectoris.

THERAPY AND FURTHER COURSE

The patient's pain was relieved by the application of nitrites which dilate the coronary arteries. This response confirmed the diagnosis. He was also told to avoid exertion.

DISCUSSION

Angina pectoris is characterized by attacks of moderate to severe chest pain originating in the heart. The attacks are usually precipitated by exertion, excitement, or a heavy meal and are relieved or diminished by rest. The pain is felt beneath the sternum and may radiate most commonly to the neck, left shoulder, or arm. The pain is customarily ex-

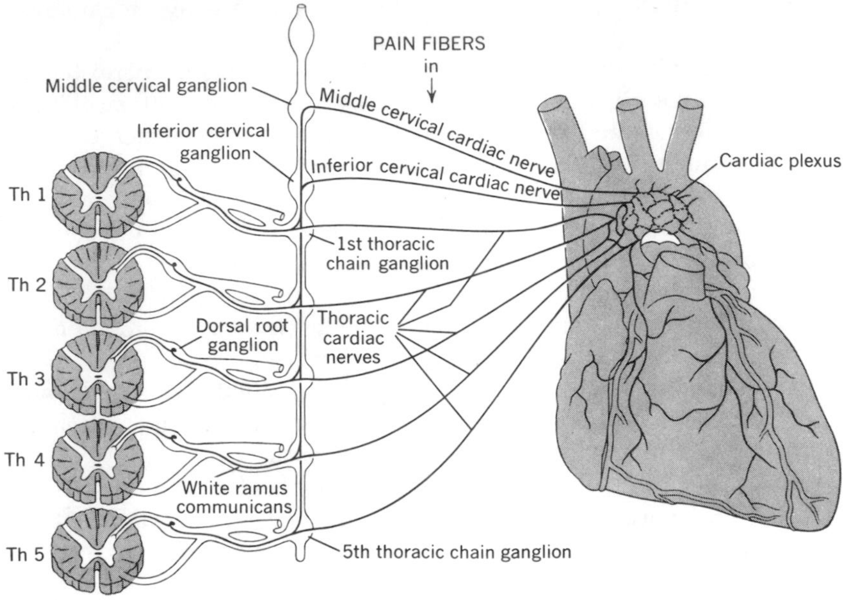

Figure 1—Pathways of cardiac pain.

plained on the basis of insufficient supply of oxygen to the heart muscle due to arteriosclerotic narrowing of the coronary arteries, particularly when the heart is required to perform increased amounts of work. However, the actual cause and exact site of origin of anginal pain are still disputed.

Pain pathways in angina pectoris

What is the anatomical pathway for pain impulses from the heart? Do all cervical cardiac nerves participate in the transmission of pain? Are the cervical cardiac nerves the only pathway for cardiac pain? Is the vagus important in the transmission of pain impulses from the heart? Where are the cell bodies of the pain fibers located? Do pain fibers return to spinal nerves via gray or white rami communicantes?

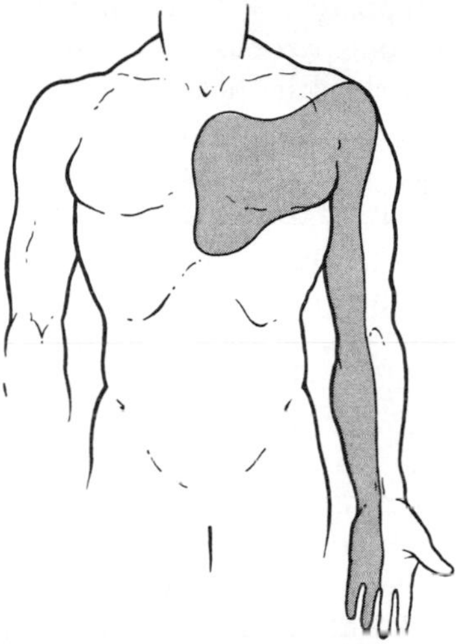

Figure 2—Typical area of pain referral in angina pectoris.

The answers to the preceding questions can be arrived at by knowledge of the anatomy of cardiac sensation. Cardiac pain impulses are received in free nerve endings in the cardiac connective tissue and the adventitia of the cardiac blood vessels. From there they travel in visceral sensory fibers through the cardiac plexus and through the middle and inferior cervical cardiac and thoracic cardiac nerves to the sympathetic chain ganglia of neck and upper thorax. From the middle and inferior cervical chain ganglia these fibers descend without synapse in the chain to upper thoracic ganglia, where other pain pathways arrive directly via thoracic cardiac nerves. From the upper four or five thoracic chain ganglia the fibers continue, again without synapse, via white rami communicantes, spinal nerves TI to TV and the corresponding dorsal roots and ganglia. Here their cell bodies are located. Central fibers from these spinal ganglia go to the upper thoracic cord segments (Fig. 1). The superior cervical cardiac nerves probably do not contain any afferent fibers and the sensory components of the vagus nerve apparently do not transmit any pain impulses from the heart, but participate in reflex actions that lower blood pressure and slow the heart beat.

The correctness of these cardiac pain pathways is confirmed by successful surgical attack of cardiac pain. The latter can be eradicated by division of the upper five thoracic dorsal spinal nerve roots on both sides. The same result will be obtained if the upper four or five thoracic chain ganglia and/or the white rami communicantes are removed or chemically blocked on both sides (Fig. 1). The left may occasionally suffice.

For physiologic reasons, cardiac pain is referred to areas of the body surface which send sensory impulses to the same segments of the cord that receive cardiac sensation, that is, mainly cervical VIII to thoracic V, with preponderance of the left side. The highest two segments listed are responsible for pain along the medial side of the arm and forearm (Fig. 2).

18 Cardiac Infarction

A 52-year-old insurance adjuster is brought to the hospital in an ambulance. His wife, who accompanied him, stated that during dinner he started to complain of excruciating chest pain in the region of the sternum. These symptoms were accompanied by nausea, vomiting, and severe shortness of breath. She also pointed out that for several years the patient has been suffering from chest pain that radiated into the left arm, particularly after physical effort or emotional upsets.

EXAMINATION AND FURTHER COURSE

On admission the patient appears in shock. His skin is ashen gray with some cyanosis (bluish tinge), and is cold and clammy. His blood pressure is low, his pulse is quite weak, and his pulse rate is 110 per minute. His respirations are noisy and gasping. On auscultation of the lungs, abnormal breath sounds are heard. His heart sounds are feeble and arrhythmic.

In spite of oxygen application, intravenous injection of circulatory stimulants, electric defibrillation and terminal cardiac massage, the patient expires within two hours after admission.

At autopsy there is found marked narrowing of both coronary arteries and many of their branches, due to atherosclerosis of the vessel wall. There is an old occlusion in the first portion of the right coronary artery and a fresh intimal hemorrhage in the anterior interventricular branch near its origin from the left coronary artery, which in combination with a fresh blood clot has completely occluded the anterior interventricular branch.

DIAGNOSIS

Sudden death due to coronary occlusion in atherosclerosis of the coronary arteries (cardiac infarction).

DISCUSSION

Ischemic heart disease, i.e. heart disease caused by insufficient blood supply to the heart muscle, is one of the most frequent conditions encountered in patients past 40 years of age and is the leading cause of death in the United States.

It is the function of the coronary arteries to carry blood to the myocardium and thus maintain its nutrition. When the lumen of the coronary arteries becomes narrowed or obliterated due to atherosclerosis of the intima, the portion of the myocardium supplied by the affected artery suffers from lack of oxygen (hypoxia) and becomes damaged. This myocardial hypoxia may result in rapid death, as happened in our patient, generally due to ventricular fibrillation. The latter condition is a cardiac arrhythmia leading to completely disorganized ventricular excitation and ineffective contraction resulting in circulatory failure and, frequently, death.

Anatomy of the coronary arteries

The decisive factor in the life of individuals with coronary atherosclerosis, then, is the state of the coronary circulation. Identify the arterial supply to the heart and give the origin of these arteries. The right and left coronary arteries are middle-sized muscular arteries that arise from the right and left aortic sinuses of the first part of the aorta just distal to the semilunar valves. The main arteries run in the epicardial fat of the atrioventricular and interventricular grooves and are partly concealed by fat and in some locations also by thin layers of ventricular myocardium, so that dissection becomes necessary for their demonstration.

To what extent does the statement that the right coronary artery supplies the right heart, and the left coronary artery the left heart, require qualification? Typically, the right coronary artery supplies the right atrium and the right ventricle with the exception of the left part of the sternocostal surface of the right ventricle, which is supplied by the left coronary artery. The left coronary artery supplies the left atrium and left ventricle with the exception of the left auricle, the posterior surface of the left atrium and the right part of the diaphragmatic aspect of the left ventricle which are supplied by the right coronary artery. What is the blood supply to the interatrial and interventricular septa where important parts of the conducting system are located? While the interatrial septum is usually supplied from the right coronary artery, both the right and left coronary vessels participate in the arterial supply of the interventricular septum through their interventricular branches, with the left commonly carrying the greater share (Fig. 2).

Are coronary arteries end-arteries?

Are coronary arteries end-arteries? What is your definition of an end-artery? End-arteries are arteries that do not anastomose (communicate) with other arteries or arterial branches of the same artery. Obstruction of such an end-artery interferes with the blood supply to that part of the organ supplied by the artery and leads to necrosis (tissue death) of that segment of the organ.

What are some vital organs that are supplied by end-arteries? The brain, liver, and kidney are nourished by arteries which do not anastomose or anastomose only to a degree insufficient to keep the segment viable that is supplied by the obstructed artery. The area of necrosis is known as an infarct. Although from the frequent occurrence of cardiac infarction we can deduce that a collateral circulation is absent, or inadequate in these cases, the branches of the coronary arteries are not true end-arteries, since numerous anastomoses take place either between the right and left coronary arteries (intercoronary anastomoses) or between branches of the same artery (intracoronary anastomoses).

Intracardiac collateral circulation

What are some of the common sites of anastomosis between the two coronary arteries? The coronary sulcus, the posterior interventricular sulcus, the area of the apex, and the interventricular septum are locations where arterial anastomoses frequently can be demonstrated (Figs. 1 and 2).

Give an example of an intracoronary anastomosis. The two main branches of the left coronary artery, the anterior interventricular and the circumflex, can often be seen to communicate around the left (obtuse) border of the heart. Normally, however, these communications, while anatomically patent, are small and functionally inactive, thus we can speak of the coronary arteries as physiologic end-arteries. In other words, the collateral circulation in the normal is usually ineffective to prevent an infarction in case of sudden interruption of the circulation. Depending on the degree of obstruction and the order and size of the obstructed arterial branch, interference with the coronary circulation may result in functional insufficiency leading to angina pectoris, i.e. cardiac pain,* or myocardial necrosis of variable extent. If, however, the occlusion of a coronary branch is slow and gradual, the anastomoses have time to enlarge and can carry an adequate circulation to the heart muscle.

How can you explain the fact that a patient who has cardiac ischemia as indicated by angina pectoris, and who survives a cardiac infarction, may be relieved of his pain afterwards? The reason for this clinically well known phenomenon is that the patient has now developed a more efficient collateral circulation than before the attack.

Sites of coronary occlusion

What are some of the sites of predilection of coronary occlusion? The most common location for coronary occlusion is the

* See previous case study.

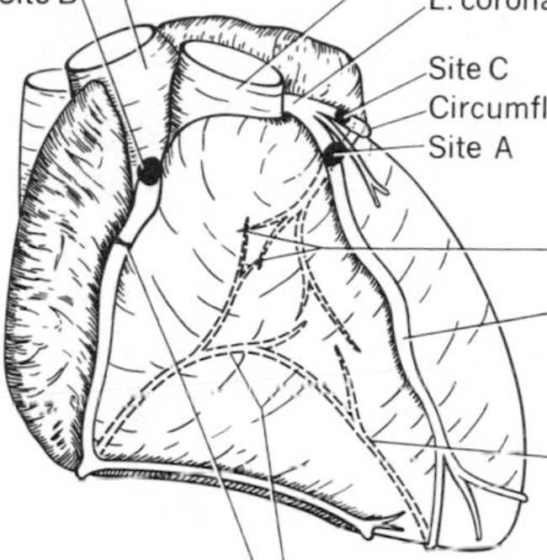

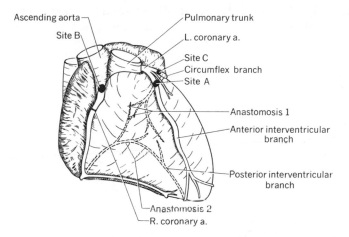

Figure 1 shows the location of two typical intercoronary anastomoses and three sites of predilection of coronary occlusion. Anastomosis (1) depicts the communication in the posterior part of the coronary sulcus between right coronary artery and circumflex branch of left coronary artery. Anastomosis (2) shows the communication in the posterior interventricular sulcus between the posterior and anterior interventricular branches of the right and left coronary arteries. Notice the three most common locations of coronary occlusion. They are in descending order of frequency: the anterior interventricular branch of the left coronary (Site A), the right coronary (Site B), and the circumflex branch of the left coronary (Site C). The occlusion occurs in all three sites, most commonly close to the origin of the vessels.

anterior interventricular branch of the left coronary (approximately 70 per cent of all cases). Next in frequency comes the right coronary, then the circumflex branch of the left coronary artery. In the vast majority of cases the occlusion involves only the proximal portion of the involved blood vessels (Fig. 1).

Variations in dominance of coronary arteries

Of great practical importance is the variation in the pattern of coronary arterial distribution from individual to individual.

Indentify the three types of distribution in terms of the dominance of one or the other of the coronary arteries. What is their respective frequency? In approximately 50 per cent the right coronary artery is the preponderant vessel which with its posterior interventricular branch supplies most of the diaphragmatic surface of both ventricles and part of the interventricular septum. In approximately 20 per cent the left coronary predominates with the posterior interventricular branch essentially being derived from the circumflex branch of the left coronary. In the remaining approximately 30 per cent there exists a balanced circulation.

Given an atherosclerotic obstruction of the left circumflex artery, which of the three types just described would be least desirable? In this case the left preponderant type would offer the greatest risk. The area of infarction would be larger than in the other types, the heart would have the least chance for development of a satisfactory collateral circulation, and the prognosis would be poorer. On the other hand, ischemic involvement of a nondominant artery would offer the best chance for development of compensatory channels.

Intramural circulation

Does all blood carried in the coronary arteries pass through the capillary bed into the cardiac veins? It is a peculiarity of the cardiac circulation that there are channels which pass from coronary arterioles, from the capillary bed, and from the cardiac veins directly into the lumen of the heart. Irregular thin-walled channels of larger than capillary size, which are called "myocardial sinusoids," also receive blood from the coronary arterioles or the capillary bed and communicate with the smallest cardiac veins (Thebesian veins) that open directly into the chambers of the heart, particularly into the atria. It has been assumed that the stream in these veins can be reversed and thus help in nourishing the ischemic myocardium in case of coronary obstruction. Some of these openings in the cardiac cavity can be seen with naked eye by inspection of the endocardial lining. They vary from pinpoint size to almost one mm in diameter.

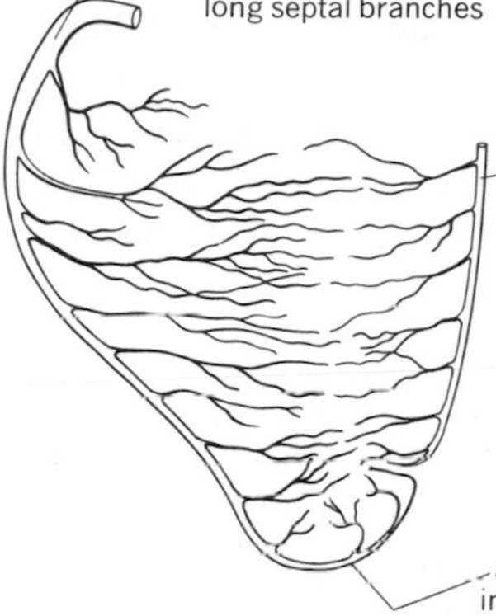

Figure 2 (modified after James and Burch) illustrates the arterial supply of the interventricular septum. Notice that in this type the anterior two-thirds of the septum are supplied by the anterior interventricular branch of the left coronary and the posterior third by the posterior interventricular branch of the right coronary. Observe the site of anastomosis between the two interventricular branches of the coronary arteries around the apex of the heart and the communications of the septal branches.

With the exception of the smallest cardiac veins, do all cardiac veins drain into the coronary sinus? The anterior cardiac veins are several smaller veins that drain part of the sternocostal surface of the right ventricle and open directly into the right atrium.

Extracardiac anastomoses

Does the coronary arterial system enter into communications with other arteries in the neighborhood and if so, how do these arteries reach the heart? How important are they for the supply of the ischemic myocardium? Anastomoses do exist between the coronary circulation and extracardiac arteries. These communications are small branches of the pericardiacophrenic and musculophrenic arteries given off by the internal thoracic artery, and of the posterior intercostal, superior phrenic, bronchial, and esophageal arteries from the aorta. They enter by way of the pericardial reflections around the major veins and arteries entering and leaving the heart. Rarely are they large enough to serve as a significant source of supply for collateral circulation in case of coronary stenosis or obstruction.

Surgical procedures utilized in production of a collateral circulation

What surgical measures have been undertaken to increase the blood supply to the ischemic heart? Experimental and clinical attempts have been made to increase the normally present and just mentioned extracardiac anastomoses of the coronary bed by obliterating the pericardiac cavity through irritants inserted into the pericardiac sac, or by scarifying the epicardial surface of the heart with the expectation that new outside vessels will invade the myocardium.

In carefully selected patients with severe angina pectoris or old coronary infarction, the left internal thoracic artery has been implanted into the myocardium of the left ventricle to provide revascularization of the ischemic heart muscle. Other sources of additional blood supply that have been utilized in the past include the implantation of the great omentum or the pectoralis major muscle.

Recent investigators have used a great saphenous vein autograft (graft from the same person) to connect the ascending aorta with the more distal portions of the right coronary artery, thus bypassing the diseased section of the artery. This approach provides instant perfusion of aortic blood into the peripheral distribution area of the right coronary artery.

Another newer technique is the direct removal of obstructing atheromatous plaques in the proximal portion of a diseased coronary artery by carbon dioxide gas, injected under pressure into the arterial wall through a small surgical opening in the artery (endarterectomy).

While the various surgical methods of revascularization of the ischemic myocardium are still under trial and subject to continuous re-evaluation and modification, surgical treatment for coronary artery disease in carefully selected cases is now an accepted method. It has a definite mortality of more than 5 per cent, but it offers hope of increased life expectancy and a useful life to a limited number of patients with coronary artery disease.

19 Coarctation of Aorta

A 28-year-old construction worker comes to the outpatient department with complaints of headache, nosebleed, occasional dizziness, and palpitations. For the past five months he also has noticed an increasing shortness of breath on exertion which, to a certain extent, has interfered with his working capacity. On routine examination six years earlier he was told that his blood pressure was elevated.

EXAMINATION

On physical examination the patient appears normally developed, in good nutritional state, and in no apparent distress. Significant findings are the following. There is considerable elevation of blood pressure in the brachial arteries, but diminished pressure in the popliteal arteries. The pulse in both femoral arteries appears quite weak and delayed as compared to the radial pulse. On percussion the left ventricle appears enlarged. On auscultation there is a systolic murmur over the heart which is also demonstrable in the interscapular area to the left of the midline.

Roentgenographic examination of the thorax shows normal lungs, but the left ventricle is hypertrophic and moderately enlarged. The aortic knob corresponding to the transitional area between arch and descending aorta is not clearly visualized and there is definite bilateral notching and erosion of the inferior margins of the posterolateral portions of ribs four to nine. The patient is admitted to the hospital.

On re-examination previous findings are confirmed and the following evidence of collateral arterial circulation of the thorax is elicited. There are pulsations visible and palpable in the interscapular area and caudal to both scapulae. Similar pulsations can be demonstrated adjacent to the clavicle and along both sides of the sternum in the area of the internal thoracic artery. On close inspection tortuous and enlarged blood vessels can be seen under the skin of the back and sides of the thorax.

On the basis of a history of hypertension and the findings of elevated blood pressure in the upper extremities and diminished pressure in the lower extremities, the weak femoral pulse, the presence of demonstrable collateral arterial circulation over the thorax, and the typical X-ray findings, a tentative diagnosis of stenosis or constriction at the isthmus of the aorta (coarctation) is made. In view of the poor prognosis in this condition, if left untreated, surgery is taken under advisement.

Preoperative roentgenographic visualization of the thoracic aorta is decided upon in order to obtain a clear picture of the anatomical condition, particularly the site, width, and length of the aortic constriction. A catheter is introduced into the radial artery against the direction of the bloodstream and pushed under fluoroscopic control as far as the ascending aorta. An X-ray opaque medium is rapidly injected and multiple roentgenographs are exposed after injection. They show a circumscribed stenosis at the typical site of the aortic isthmus beyond the origin of the left subclavian artery. The prestenotic segment of the aorta is somewhat wider than normal, the brachiocephalic trunk and the left common carotid and subclavian arteries are also moderately enlarged. The poststenotic segment is likewise, but only faintly visualized immediately after injection, proving that the obstruction of the aorta is incomplete. The following greatly widened and tortuous arteries are demonstrated by opacification as part of the collateral circulation. The right and left internal thoracic arteries are seen to anastomose with the inferior epigastric arteries, an enlarged subscapular artery and a few tortuous posterior intercostal arteries are also visualized.

DIAGNOSIS

Circumscribed stenosis of the aortic isthmus with well developed collateral circulation.

THERAPY

In view of the anatomical findings of a circumscribed obstruction at the typical site, grafting or the utilization of a vascular prosthesis is ruled out, and an end-to-end anastomosis after resection of the stenotic portion is planned.

Under general endotracheal anesthesia the aorta is approached from the left side of the chest where the fourth rib is removed and the thorax entered through the bed of the resected rib. Several enlarged and tortuous vessels of the chest wall are encountered and doubly ligated. The aorta is mobilized above and below the stenosed area, starting just distal to the left subclavian artery. Here several dilated and fragile posterior intercostal arteries are seen and ligated. The ligamentum arteriosum is ligated and divided. After the aorta is sufficiently freed, it is clamped on either side of the constricted portion with special non-crushing clamps and the area of coarctation is excised. Enough vascular tissue is resected to provide for normal caliber at the site of the anastomosis. Then the cut ends of the aorta are approximated, everted, and sutured together so that the interior of the vessel is covered everywhere by intima. The clamps are slowly opened and the suture lines checked for leaks. The chest wall is closed, leaving a catheter behind for drainage.

The excised specimen shows that the lumen of the aorta at the constricted site consists only of a small opening not more than 2 mm. in diameter and narrower than was expected from the outside appearance of the aorta. The obstruction in the interior of the aorta is due to a diaphragm-like infolding of the media with some secondary intimal thickening. The aortic end of the ligamentum arteriosum, which was removed with the narrowed segment of the aorta, is non-patent.

FURTHER COURSE

During the operation and postoperatively the patient was given blood transfusions. Postoperatively, he had some fever and was given antibiotics. After this the temperature slowly returned to normal. The patient was gradually allowed to get up. He was dismissed from the hospital three weeks after the operation. During this period pulsations in the femoral artery gradually increased in intensity. There was also a gradual diminution of blood pressure in the upper extremity and concomitant increase to normal in the lower. The patient was seen six months and one year after the operation. He was well satisfied with the result and had returned to his former work. His blood pressure in the upper and lower extremities remained normal.

DISCUSSION

We are dealing here with a congenital cardiovascular anomaly, which occurs with a frequency of one in 1500 to 2000 of all autopsies. It is four or five times more common in males than in females. Coarctation (from the Latin *coarctare,* to constrict) is a pathologic condition in which the lumen of the aortic arch or of the descending aorta just beyond the arch is significantly constricted on a congenital basis.

What is your definition of the term "isthmus of the aorta?" It is that portion of the aortic arch between the left subclavian artery and the ductus arteriosus. It is normally constricted at birth but enlarges soon thereafter as the duct becomes obliterated. This is also the typical site of a diffuse type of coarctation of the aorta in the infant, in which case the ductus arteriosus often remains patent. More common is the type in which clinical signs and symptoms become apparent only during adult life and in which the constriction is more circumscribed and located at or just beyond the point of entrance of the ductus arteriosus (or ligament) as in our case (Fig. 1). Other variants also occur, yet rarely as, for example, an aortic stenosis proximal (not distal) to the origin of the left subclavian artery.

Cause of coarctation

Can you offer any explanation for the occurrence of congenital coarctation of the aorta? The cause of the condition was thought to be an extension into the aorta of the obliterative

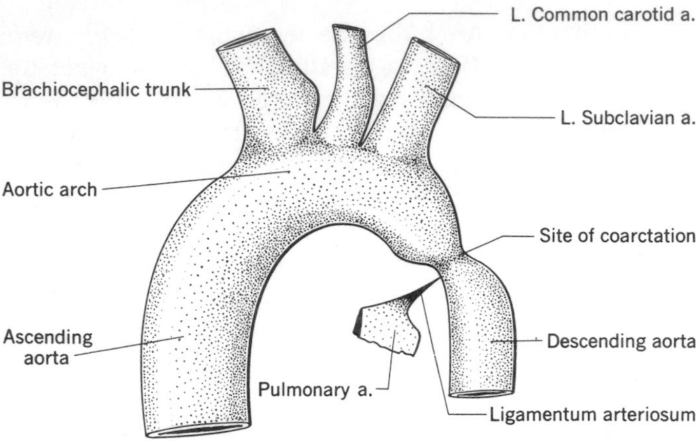

Figure 1 shows coarctation of aorta beyond the origin of the left subclavian artery at the site of attachment of the ligamentum arteriosum. Aortic arch and its branches are dilated.

process which occludes the ductus arteriosus. This view seems hardly tenable if one realizes that coarctation frequently occurs in the absence of obliteration of the duct. Other explanations offered are traction on the aortic wall with infolding of the media due to the pull of the ductus arteriosus, the dimensions of which do not keep step with the growth of the aorta. A 1962 edition of a scholarly monograph by R. A. Willis on *The Borderland of Embryology and Pathology* regards the mode of genesis of the malformation as obscure, although probably related to the involution of the ductus arteriosus. From what primitive aortic arch is the latter derived? The ductus arteriosus represents the dorsal part of the left sixth arch.

Explanation of signs and symptoms

How do you explain the clinical symptoms of our patient, consisting of headache, nosebleed, and dizziness, in the light of the anatomical picture of a circumscribed stenosis of the aorta? The complaints of our patient are due to increased blood pressure in the prestenotic portion of the aorta and its branches.

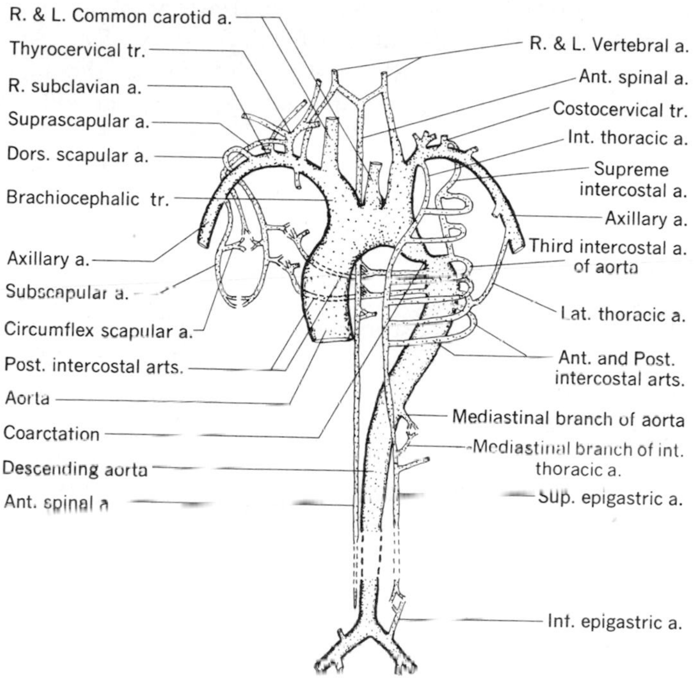

Figure 2 shows various sites of collateral circulation in a case of aortic coarctation.

This is most likely caused by the additional resistance offered to the propulsion of the blood at the site of the stenosis. It is also borne out by the objective finding of hypertension in both brachial arteries present in our patient. As a result of the greatly increased intra-arterial pressure in the prestenotic portion of the aorta, the aortic arch and its branches are enlarged and the left ventricle becomes hypertrophied and dilated. This leads to gradual failure of the heart with respiratory distress on exertion; this is also present in our patient. Are there clinical signs of decreased pressure in the post-stenotic part of the aorta and its branches? Hypotension was demonstrated in the popliteal artery and was also indicated by the weakened pulse in the femoral artery. Where do you normally feel the pulse of the femoral artery? The pulse is elicited by palpating rather deeply inferior to the inguinal ligament, midway between anterior superior iliac spine and symphysis pubis.

Collateral circulation

What features in the clinical picture of our patient demonstrate the presence of a collateral circulation which allows blood to bypass the constriction and to which can be ascribed the survival of the patient (Fig. 2)? In addition to the direct radiographic evidence of enlarged and tortuous vessels in the region of the thoracic wall, we find visible and palpable pulsations in the interscapular area and all along the thoracic wall, particularly at both sides of the sternum. On close inspection dilated arteries can also be seen under the skin of the thorax. Is there evidence that coarctation in our case is not complete? Direct opacification of the thoracic aorta demonstrated immediate, but faint, filling of the poststenotic area.

These then are the sources of arterial blood in the poststenotic portion of the aorta and its branches: direct filling through a narrowed aperture in the aorta at the constricted site, and an indirect discharge of blood into the peripheral distribution area of the abdominal aorta through well-developed collateral arterial channels. Fortunately for the patient there are in this location of the arterial obstruction ample communicating channels available which permit the development of a collateral flow around the partial occlusion.

What are these vessels? For purposes of classification they can be divided into several groups: (1) The scapular and cervical anastomosis. Scapular and cervical branches from the subclavian and axillary arteries carry blood from above the obstruction to posterior intercostal arteries coming off the aorta below the obstruction. Identify these branches. They are the transverse and deep cervical, the suprascapular and dorsal scapular arteries, derived directly or indirectly from the subclavian artery and the subscapular and its circumflex scapular branch of the axillary artery. Some of these channels could be seen or their pulsation felt in our patient. (2) The internal thoracic anastomosis. This was clearly demonstrated in our case on the opacified roentgenogram of the aortic circulation. The internal thoracic artery, a branch of the subclavian artery, anastomoses by way of its anterior intercostal arteries with the posterior intercostal aortic branches, and its musculophrenic and mediastinal branches communicate with phrenic and mediastinal branches of the descending aorta. Finally, one of its two important terminal branches, the superior epigastric artery, anastomoses with the inferior epigastric from the external iliac, thus bypassing the coarcted area of the aorta. (3) The intercostal anastomosis. This has already been referred to in relation to the communications between the anterior and posterior intercostal branches of the internal thoracic artery and aorta respectively. It also includes the communications between the highest intercostal artery from the costocervical trunk of the subclavian artery, and the posterior intercostal artery for the third space from the descending aorta. (4) The spinal anastomosis. The anterior spinal artery derived from the vertebral artery, a branch of the subclavian, communicates with segmental spinal branches of the posterior intercostals from the descending aorta, from the lumbar and lateral sacral arteries and thus establishes a further collateral channel in coarctation of the aorta. Here it is often dilated and tortuous.

One roentgenographic finding demonstrable on routine chest films is caused by the development of the collateral circulation just described and remains as the single most important radiologic sign of aortic coarctation. Identify it. It is the notching and erosion of the bodies of the ribs in the area of the costal grooves, and is caused by the sometimes greatly enlarged posterior intercostal arteries. These dilated arteries may occasionally cause difficulties for the surgeon since they often become quite friable. Some of them may have to be ligated and excised as in our case.

What is the clinical significance of the delayed appearance of the femoral pulse in our case? It proves that probably the major portion of the blood coursing through the femoral artery arrived in the artery by way of devious collateral channels rather than directly through the stenotic area. Does the presence of a clearly demonstrable pulse in the more caudally located arterial channels in the leg, such as the posterior tibial artery at the medial side of the ankle or in the dorsal pedis artery, rule out aortic coarctation? It does not prove the absence of aortic obstruction since a well-developed collateral circulation may keep these arteries well supplied with blood. How do you explain the systolic murmur demonstrable over the cardiac and left interscapular areas? It is due to obstruction to the free flow of blood from the left ventricle to the descending aorta at the time of ventricular contraction.

Causes of fatal outcome in untreated cases

A final question needs to be discussed. Why is dangerous surgery, which may on occasion be fatal, indicated in this case when the clinical complaints of the patient are relatively insignificant? If left unoperated, three-fourths of these cases will die before the age of forty. The average life expectancy of all cases of coarctation is thirty-five years. What is the cause of death in these cases? The harmful effects of coarctation are derived from the hypertension in the upper part of the body. This may eventually lead to cardiac failure and death. The prestenotic area of the aorta will dilate and may rupture. Cerebral vessels derived from vertebral and internal carotid arteries likewise dilate as a result of the hypertension and may also rupture, leading to fatal cerebral hemorrhage. Finally, bacterial infection may occur at the site of coarctation or at a bicuspid aortic valve, a complication that is a frequent accompaniment of aortic coarctation.

20 Obstruction of Superior Vena Cava

A 57-year-old man is admitted to the hospital because of recurrent nosebleed and progressive shortness of breath. The bleeding from the nose started three and one-half months earlier and required two admissions to the hospital. The shortness of breath began three years prior to admission and was particularly noticeable on exertion. Chronic cough gradually developed.

For the past twenty-four years the patient has noticed a gradual appearance of distended tortuous veins over the anterior part of the chest wall and at that time began to complain of dizziness, especially on arising and bending over. The face appeared puffy with a bluish hue, which became worse when he reclined or bent forward. His collar size increased although he did not gain any weight. The patient recalls that prior to the development of these veins he had many bad furuncles and carbuncles on the trunk and in both axillae, extending over years.

EXAMINATION

On examination the patient shows cyanosis of the face and neck. With the patient in the supine position the cyanosis deepens. The eyes are prominent and the eyelids slightly swollen. There are numerous prominent tortuous superficial

The actual case is taken from a paper by L. B. Rose: Obstruction of the Superior Vena Cava of Twenty-five Years' Duration, J.A.M.A., 150:12; 1198-1200, 1952.

veins over the neck, both arms, axillae, and anterior chest wall. Numerous veins cross the anterior costal margins and continue down over the abdomen toward the pubic area. The entire trunk is covered with large acne-type skin eruptions and numerous old healed scars of previous skin lesions. In contrast to the upper extremities, the skin of the lower extremities is of normal color.

Further physical examination reveals signs of chronic pulmonary emphysema (overdistention of the lungs), otherwise the internal organs are normal.

X-ray study of the chest shows a widening of the mediastinal shadow in the region of the right upper mediastinum and a group of heavily calcified lymph nodes lying against the right side of the trachea down to the level of the bifurcation. Roentgenograms of the chest following injection of a contrast medium into the cubital vein reveal that the widening of the upper mediastinum is composed mainly of abnormal veins. The termination of the right subclavian vein appears to be constricted and accompanied by numerous collateral channels. Complete obstruction is present in the right brachiocephalic vein caudal to its formation by the confluence of internal jugular and subclavian veins. No contrast medium enters the heart during the X-ray exposure, but is diverted to maximally dilated and tortuous collateral veins in and over the upper part of the thorax. The medium is seen to enter an enlarged internal thoracic vein which descends and joins with greatly dilated abdominal veins. There is no filling of the terminal portion of the azygos vein. Studies of venous pressure show three times the normal pressure in the veins of the upper extremities, while the pressure in the veins of the lower extremities is normal.

DIAGNOSIS

Obstruction of superior vena cava.

DISCUSSION

The progressive shortness of breath and the cough of the patient can be ascribed to pulmonary emphysema, resulting from chronic bronchitis and degenerative changes in the lungs. These symptoms are apparently not connected with the other outstanding findings.

The swelling of the face, the bleeding from the nose, the cyanosis, and the increased pressure in the veins of upper extremity, as well as the distention and tortuosity of the veins of neck, arms, and upper trunk are due to an obstruction of the venous channels which drain the blood from the upper part of the body. Since the obstruction is of such long standing (twenty-five years), and based on the clinical findings and X-ray studies, a benign cause has to be assumed. In view of the history of severe skin infections of the chest wall extending over several years, the obstruction can reasonably be ascribed to thrombosis (clotting of blood) in mediastinal veins originating from an inflammation of these veins. What main veins are involved? The right brachiocephalic vein and the superior vena cava are definitely involved. Why does distention of the visible veins increase in the supine position and on bending forward? Keep in mind the direction of the blood flow and the absence of valves in the veins of the mediastinum.

The calcification of mediastinal lymph nodes in the area of the obstructed veins furthermore suggests the presence of inflammatory changes in these nodes caused by infection of the adjacent areas. Thus, the combination of chronic inflammation of the mediastinal lymph nodes with scarring and compression of the veins of the mediastinum and of clotting inside these veins resulted in obstruction of the right brachiocephalic vein and the superior vena cava. Clinical tests and the roentgenogram also indicate obstruction of the azygos vein at the site of its termination (Fig. 1).

The most common cause of obstruction of the superior vena cava, in addition to the two factors effective here, are neoplasms, either pressing upon or invading the superior vena cava. Circumscribed enlargement (aneurysm) of what large artery in the neighborhood of the superior vena cava would also be apt to compress the vein? An aneurysm of the ascending aorta could easily lead to compression of the superior vena cava.

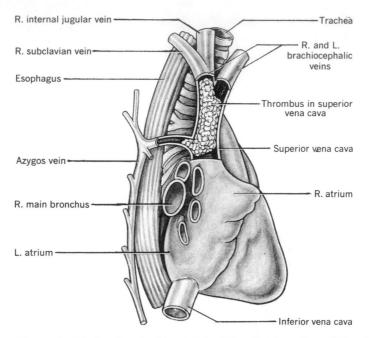

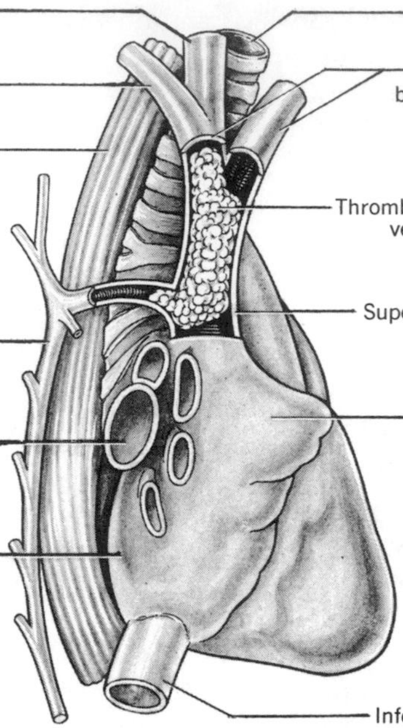

Figure 1—Obstruction by blood clot of the distal portion of the right brachiocephalic vein, the superior vena cava, and the terminal part of the azygos vein.

Collateral venous pathways in obstruction of the superior vena cava

What collateral venous channels are available in this case where the distal portion of the right brachiocephalic vein, the superior vena cava, and the termination of the azygos vein are obstructed? How is the return of venous blood to the right atrium from the upper part of the body accomplished? Keep in mind that in this case where the termination of the azygos vein is also obstructed, all blood that normally drains into the superior vena cava has to return to the heart by way of the inferior vena cava (Fig. 2).

The visible dilatation and tortuosity of the superficial veins of neck, arms, and trunk indicate that these channels are involved in the bypass to the inferior vena cava. They comprise

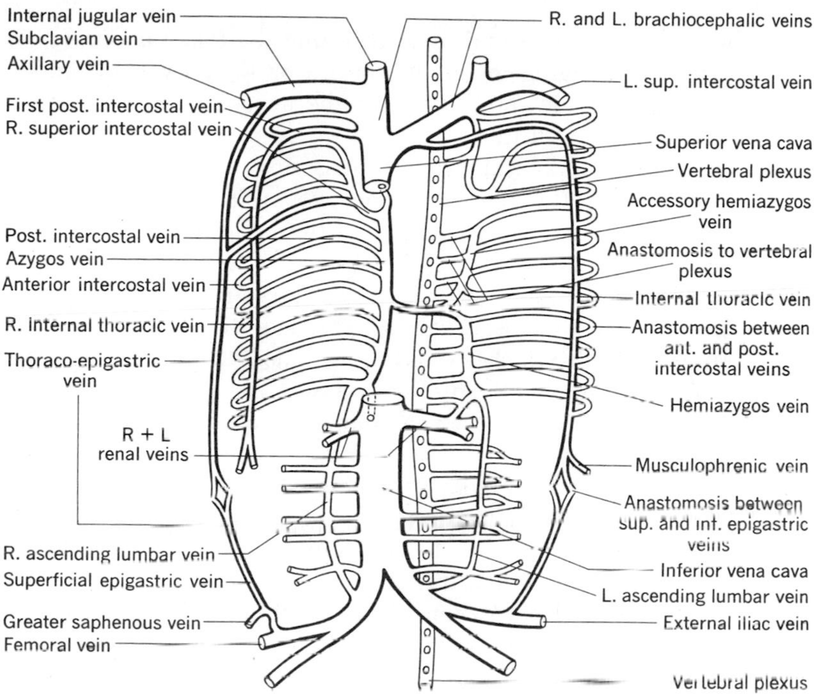

Figure 2—Diagrammatic representation of the four main collateral systems effective in obstruction of the superior vena cava. Notice (1) the superficial venous system, represented by the thoraco-epigastric vein, (2) the internal thoracic system with the anastomosis between superior and inferior epigastric veins, (3) the vertebral plexus, and (4) the azygos route and its anastomoses with other systems.

anastomoses between the veins of the thoracic wall, that normally drain into the axillary and internal thoracic veins, and tributaries of the femoral vein. One of the numerous veins belonging to this group is designated as thoracoepigastric vein. What named veins, draining eventually into the superior and inferior vena cava respectively, does this vein connect? It connects the lateral thoracic vein cranially with the superficial epigastric vein caudally. The lateral thoracic vein drains into the axillary vein and the superficial epigastric vein drains into the great saphenous and through it into the femoral vein (Fig. 2). Veins belonging to this group are particularly involved in the bypass, if the termination of the azygos vein is also obstructed, as in our case.

A second collateral system bypassing the obstruction is represented by the internal thoracic venous system. Here again reversal of blood flow is facilitated by the absence or scarcity of valves. Named communicating vessels of this system are represented by the superior epigastric vein, musculophrenic vein, anterior intercostal veins, and perforating and mammary branches. With which named veins belonging to the inferior caval system do these veins anastomose? These veins which are all tributaries of the internal thoracic veins, anastomose directly or indirectly with the inferior epigastric veins which drain into the external iliac veins (Fig. 2).

A third channel is represented by the vertebral plexus of veins. Where in relation to the spinal column is this plexus located? Do the veins draining into this plexus anastomose with previously listed veins? What anatomical feature in this plexus would facilitate reversal of the bloodstream? The vertebral plexus of veins comprises an aggregate of veins extending from the head to the sacrum on the outside of the spinal column anteriorly and posteriorly as well as inside the vertebral canal. These veins are characterized not only by rich anastomoses with segmental veins, such as the intercostals, but also by longitudinal anastomoses and by cross-communications between right and left, and by anastomoses from inside the vertebral canal to the outside. Reversal of the bloodstream is facilitated by the absence of valves in this plexus (Fig. 2).

Azygos route

The azygos route, although its normal drainage into the superior vena cava is blocked here, can contribute to the collateral circulation through reversal of its blood flow and by virtue of the fact that it receives important segmental tributaries from the thoracic wall and from the other bypassing systems mentioned previously. What are these segmental tributaries? How is the azygos vein formed? Locate its anastomoses with the internal thoracic and vertebral routes. Usually the azygos vein is formed by the confluence of the right ascending lumbar and subcostal veins. It frequently also connects directly with the inferior vena cava. It receives its segmental venous contributions through the lower right posterior intercostal veins directly and through the right superior intercostal vein indirectly. It also receives left segmental contributions commonly through the hemiazygos and accessory hemiazygos veins. All these intercostal veins are the channels of anastomosis with the internal thoracic and vertebral routes (Fig. 2).

What additional collateral channels would be available if the superior vena cava were obstructed above the point of entrance of the azygos vein? One has to realize that in case of patency (openness) of the azygos vein, the latter would be capable of carrying blood to the lower part of the superior vena cava, in addition to the previously mentioned bypasses to the inferior vena cava.

If, instead of the superior vena cava, the inferior vena cava were obstructed, could the same veins also be employed to channel blood to the superior vena cava? This would be possible by simple reversal of the blood flow in the previously listed channels.

THERAPY AND FURTHER COURSE

The chronic bronchitis and emphysema improved under drug treatment and respiratory exercises. The venous obstruction continued to cause mild symptoms.

21 Cancer of the Esophagus

A 53-year-old carpenter is admitted to the hospital as an emergency. He has severe shortness of breath (dyspnea) and great difficulty in swallowing (dysphagia). The patient states that for the past six months he has suffered increasing difficulty and pain in swallowing. He has had to subsist on a liquid diet and has lost thirty pounds of weight. His shortness of breath has been present for the past three months. From time to time he has severe coughing spells, his sputum is blood-tinged, and occasionally he brings up as much as a cupful of blood. He states that for the last few weeks he has become quite hoarse. He also has noticed a tumorous swelling on his right shoulder which is painful on motion.

EXAMINATION

On examination the patient appears quite emaciated and in great distress. Laryngoscopic examination reveals the left vocal fold in semi-abducted position on respiration and phonation. His face is dark purple in color and he suffers from labored respiration. His pulse is rapid and his temperature is 101°.

X-ray examination of the chest shows widening of the mediastinum with destruction of the lateral half of the right clavicle corresponding to the soft tissue tumor in this area. Brief fluoroscopic examination of the esophagus with radiopaque barium

This presentation is based on an actual case history and autopsy report at the University Hospital, Oklahoma City.

demonstrates an obstruction at the level of the bifurcation of the trachea.

FURTHER COURSE

Patient was put on oxygen and narcotics and was given intravenous fluids. On the fourth day he became comatose and expired.

At autopsy a large cauliflower-like tumor was found in the esophagus that obstructed the lumen of the esophagus. The esophagus above the obstruction was greatly dilated. At the level of the tracheal bifurcation the mass had perforated into the trachea which showed an ulcerous communication with the esophagus (Fig. 1 and 2). The tumor mass surrounded and compressed the trachea over an area 3 cm. in length. The left recurrent laryngeal nerve was likewise embedded in the mass. The mediastinal lymph nodes particularly in the posterior mediastinum were greatly enlarged and tumorous and adhered to each other. The dependent portions of both lungs showed signs of bronchopneumonia. There were nodular metastases of varying size in both lungs and scattered over the visceral pleura. There also were round tumor masses in the liver. On microscopic examination the area of destruction of the right clavicle was found to be a cancerous metastasis.

DIAGNOSIS

Cancer of the esophagus with obstruction and perforation into the trachea and metastatic involvement of regional lymph nodes, of lungs and pleura, liver, and clavicle.

DISCUSSION

We are dealing here with the terminal course of an esophageal cancer which has obstructed the esophagus at one of the most common sites of esophageal cancer, that is, the level of the tracheal bifurcation. The preferred sites of esophageal cancer correspond to the physiologic constrictions of the esophagus.

Where are these located? One is found at the beginning of the organ in the neck at the level of the cricoid cartilage. The second is at the level of the bifurcation of the trachea and the third at the site of the esophageal passage through the diaphragm. Other narrowings are often described at the level of the aortic arch and just below the bifurcation where the left bronchus crosses the esophagus. The dilatation of the esophagus above the obstruction, which is found in our case, is common in cases of esophageal stenosis and represents the result of mechanical stretching of the organ by the ingested food and liquid above the site of the impasse.

Topographic anatomy of the esophagus as applied to cancer

The complications of the esophageal cancer caused by invasion of organs and structures in its neighborhood are exemplified in our case by the compression of and break-through into the trachea and the paralysis of the left recurrent laryngeal nerve. What coat is lacking in the wall of the esophagus that in most of the other portions of the gastrointestinal tract serves as at least a temporary barrier to cancerous invasion of the neighborhood? The esophagus does not have a serosal coat and is separated from the trachea by only a small amount of areolar tissue, explaining the frequent involvement of the trachea in esophageal cancer. The compression of the trachea by the tumor mass explains the severe dyspnea and cyanosis (purple discoloration due to deficient oxygenation of the blood by the lungs) of the patient. The invasion and ulcerous penetration of the trachea caused the bronchopneumonia, the tracheal hemorrhages, and the blood-tinged sputum mentioned previously. What arteries supply the trachea and esophagus at the level of the bifurcation, branches of which were eroded by the cancer in our case? Bronchial arteries and direct visceral branches of the thoracic aorta are responsible for the blood supply of the two tubes.

How do you explain the paralysis of the left recurrent laryngeal nerve, which resulted in the hoarseness and change in position of the left vocal fold as revealed by laryngoscopic

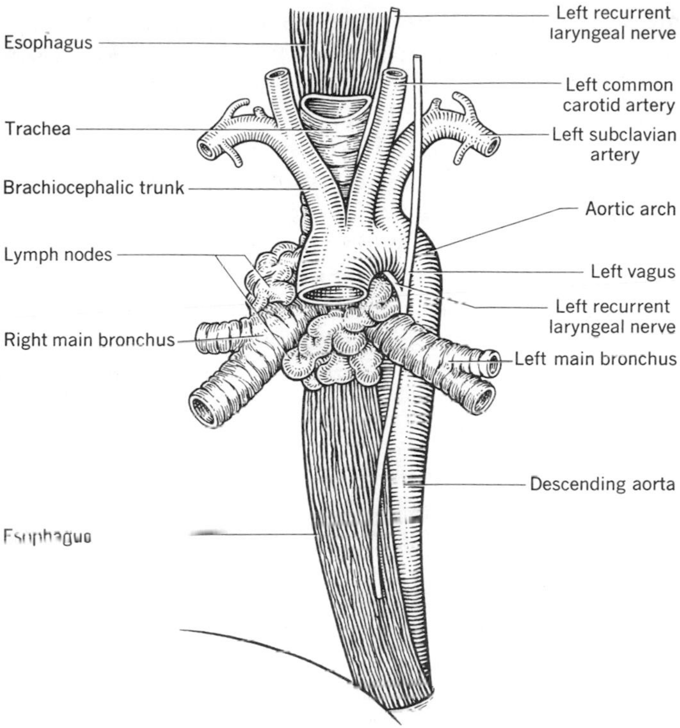

Figure 1—Anterior view of esophagus, trachea, and aorta showing the changing relationship of the aorta to the esophagus and the course of the left recurrent laryngeal nerve in relation to aorta, trachea, and esophagus. Notice the enlarged and cancerous lymph nodes and the dilatation of the upper thoracic portion of the esophagus.

examination? The left recurrent laryngeal nerve arises from the vagus where the latter passes over the left (lateral) aspect of the aortic arch. It then winds below the arch to gain its medial aspect and from there runs upward in a gutter-like groove on the left side of the trachea and esophagus (Fig. 1). As frequently occurs in esophageal cancer, the mass compressed the nerve and paralyzed it. What is the function of the recurrent laryngeal nerves in the larynx? They supply all laryngeal muscles with the exception of the cricothyroid muscle. Paralysis of the nerve immobilizes the vocal fold of that side and puts it in a semi-abducted position. Does the recurrent laryngeal nerve also send sensory fibers to the larynx? It supplies the mucous membrane of the larynx below the vocal folds. Why is the left recurrent laryngeal nerve more frequently paralyzed than the right in cancer of the esophagus? This is due to the difference in the course of the two nerves, with the right entering into relationship only with the cervical portion of the esophagus.

Knowledge of the anatomical relations of the thoracic esophagus will allow us to identify other structures and organs frequently penetrated by the growing cancer. Thus, in addition to trachea and main bronchi, the pleural cavity, the lungs, the aorta, and the pericardium and heart may be invaded. Due to the closer relationship of the left bronchus to the esophagus this bronchus is more frequently involved than the right. On the other hand, it is the right mediastinal pleura which is more apt to insinuate itself between esophagus and aorta forming a retro-esophageal recess; it is therefore more commonly involved than the left in the pleural spread of esophageal cancer. Perforation into the aorta may lead to immediate fatal hemorrhage. Remember that in the posterior mediastinum the aorta is at first on the left side and then posterior to the esophagus, in which relationship they pass through the diaphragm. "The thickness of the pericardium and esophagus is all that intervenes between the wall of the left atrium and the food you swallow" (Grant). Consequently, the left atrium is the chamber of the heart that may be infiltrated by cancerous growth from the esophagus (Fig. 2).

Lymphatic spread of esophageal cancer

Cancer does not only spread locally by invasive growth to the surrounding tissues and organs. More important even for the final outcome is the penetration of the lymphatic and vascular channels which disseminate clusters of tumor cells (tumor emboli) to all parts of the body. This dissemination is well exemplified in our case. Our patient had large masses of can-

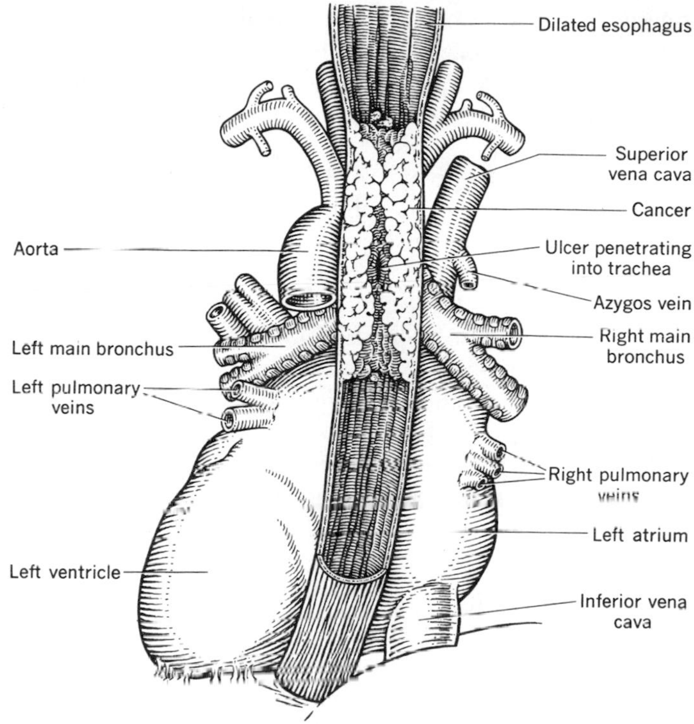

Figure 2—Posterior view of the esophagus with the esophagus partly opened. The extensive obstructing cancer is shown as well as the erosion into the trachea and the enlargement of the esophagus above the obstruction. Notice the close relationship of the esophagus to the left atrium.

cerous lymph nodes demonstrable on the X-ray film in the posterior mediastinum. These, together with periesophageal lymph nodes adjacent to the organ and tracheobronchial nodes, represent the area of regional lymph drainage from the middle portions of the esophagus. We have to visualize that the primary tumor invaded the lymph capillaries in the mucosa and spread from there by way of the lymph vessels in the esophageal musculature to the regional lymph nodes. Lymphatic metastases from the esophageal cancer may reach these regional lymph nodes first and then, due to rich lymphatic anastomoses, may spread to nodes located at considerable distance, ascending as far as the neck or descending to lymph nodes in the abdomen around the celiac artery.

The common involvement of lungs and pleura, which was also present in our case, might be explained on the basis of direct spread of the primary cancer. More likely though is retrograde dissemination of the cancer through the lymphatics of lung and pleura from the cancerous tracheobronchial lymph nodes. It should also be kept in mind that all lymph and with it cancerous emboli finally reach the venous circulation through the termination of the thoracic and right lymphatic ducts in the venous angles of the neck. Thus, lymphatic spread, if not arrested by surgery or radiation, in the end brings cancerous fragments into the venous circulation and from there to the lungs which are a common site of metastasis.

Venous spread of esophageal cancer

Invasion of the esophageal veins at the site of the tumor must also be assumed to have taken place and with it spread of cancerous emboli along venous channels. Where do the veins of the esophagus drain? The wall of the esophagus is an important site of anastomoses between systemic veins that drain blood by way of the azygos and hemiazygos veins into the superior vena cava and veins that are tributaries of the portal system, such as the lower esophageal veins. The latter drain into the left gastric (coronary) vein. Cancerous invasion of and spread via the lower esophageal veins explains the metastatic involvement of the liver in our case.

If some of these cancerous emboli were small enough to be transported by way of the portal vein and its branches through the sinusoids of the liver, how would they ultimately arrive in the capillary bed of the lung? They would pass through hepatic veins into the inferior vena cava, the right atrium and ventricle, and from there through the pulmonary arteries into the pulmonary circulation. On the other hand, how would spread via the esophageal veins draining into the azygos vein reach the lungs? The azygos vein empties into the superior vena cava which drains into the right heart. Thus dissemination of the cancer through superior and inferior venae cavae might readily be an additional explanation of metastatic involvement of the lungs.

Arterial spread of esophageal cancer

The final pathway for metastasis from and through the lung is the general arterial circulation. Is this terminal phase of cancerous spread exemplified in our case? The involvement of the right clavicle can be explained only on the basis of an arterial metastasis. How did the cancer, that in one way or other had reached the venous circulation, locate in the nutritional artery of the clavicle? After breaking into the tributaries of the pulmonary veins, clusters of cancer cells must have passed to and through the left heart, aorta, and its branches to the nutritional vessel of the clavicle.

In summarizing we see that, as is so often the case in terminal cancer, the growth in this patient utilized all available channels for dissemination through the body: direct invasion of structures in the neighborhood, such as the trachea and recurrent laryngeal nerve; lymphatic spread to regional lymph nodes and lungs; venous spread to the liver and possibly lungs and pleura; and arterial dissemination to the clavicle.

Abdominal and Pelvic Viscera

22 Biliary Colic–Cholecystectomy

A 46-year-old farm woman was brought by ambulance to the hospital in acute distress with symptoms of severe pain in the right upper abdominal region. In the past she has had repeated attacks of severe pain in the right upper quadrant of the abdomen, frequently following a heavy meal. These attacks were accompanied by nausea and vomiting. She suffers from indigestion and "gas pain on her stomach," particularly after eating fatty foods and eggs.

EXAMINATION

The patient is a short, stocky and rather obese woman, who has had five deliveries and two miscarriages. She complains of severe, sharp, and constant pain that started in the epigastric and umbilical regions and then became localized in the right hypochondriac area. The pain radiates around the right chest to and below the inferior angle of the scapula. She is nauseated and vomits occasionally. There is marked tenderness and some rigidity in the right hypochondriac region. She has moderate fever. Her white blood cell count is elevated. On X-ray examination without the use of contrast medium there are seen multiple calcified stones in the area of the gall bladder.

DIAGNOSIS

Biliary colic; chronic calculous cholecystitis (inflammation of the gall bladder accompanied by stone formation) with acute exacerbation.

THERAPY AND FURTHER COURSE

The patient is given opiates for her pain and prepared for surgery.

Under general anesthesia the abdominal wall is opened by a subcostal incision that begins at the tip of the xiphoid process and is directed laterally and downward, paralleling the costal margin about two fingerbreadths caudal to it. After the anterior layer of the rectus sheath has been split, the rectus is cut in a direction paralleling the skin incision. The incision is continued laterally through the external oblique, the internal oblique, and the transversus muscles in a direction paralleling the skin incision. The posterior layer of the rectus sheath is likewise divided, as is the transversalis fascia, the extraperitoneal fat, and the peritoneum. During this procedure an attempt is made to preserve the pair of intercostal nerves as they are seen within the rectus sheath deep to the rectus muscle by retracting them out of the way.

After the peritoneal cavity has been opened, it is explored with one hand with particular attention to the stomach, duodenum and transverse colon, and dome of the liver. The organs in question are found to be free from gross pathology in our case, except for numerous adhesions in the neighborhood of the gall bladder. The gall bladder is identified and on palpation is found to be thick-walled, contracted by scarring, and seems to contain numerous hard stones. The operative field is walled-off with gauze pads.

The surgeon then introduces his finger into the foramen epiploicum and between this finger and the thumb palpates the common bile duct within the lesser omentum for evidence of stones and of thickening and dilatation. In our case the common duct appears normal. With the gall bladder being retracted out of the way by its fundus, an incision is made into the lesser omentum, close to its free border. By blunt dissection the cystic duct is exposed at its junction with the neck of the gall bladder and doubly clamped and divided. Next the cystic artery is identified, doubly ligated, and likewise divided between ligatures. The peritoneal attachment of the gall bladder to the liver is incised to free the gall bladder, and the gall bladder is separated from its bed by blunt and sharp dissection. After the gall bladder has been dissected free, it is turned upward and resected.

The gall bladder bed is covered by suturing the peritoneal flaps over it. The field is inspected for bleeding and a small drain is placed into the subhepatic area. The incisions are closed in layers.

The gall bladder bed is covered by suturing the peritoneal of its walls and an inflamed mucosa. It is filled with numerous small multifaceted stones.

Postoperatively the patient is given intravenous glucose and saline solution. Gastric suction through a tube is applied for two days. In the absence of leakage of bile, the drain is removed after three days. The patient is permitted out of bed for a few minutes on the first postoperative day. This is gradually increased every day, and so is her diet after the suction has been discontinued. The further postoperative course is uneventful and the patient is discharged from the hospital on the tenth postoperative day.

DISCUSSION

We are dealing with a patient who, by virtue of her sex, age, obesity, and numerous past pregnancies, offers the most common constitutional features of a person prone to gall bladder disease.

While it is not quite clear whether gallstones form as a result of infection or metabolic disturbances, the latter seems more likely. These metabolic deviations, in conjunction with stagnation of bile in the gall bladder through spasm or organic obstruction of the duct system, encourage the formation of gallstones of various types. Later on, the accumulation of gallstones, combined with frequently superimposed secondary infection, results in an acute or chronic inflammation of the gall bladder with the classical symptoms of epigastric pain, "gas on the stomach," indigestion, nausea, and vomiting, particularly after fatty meals. The latter symptoms are due to reflex spasms of the pylorus and probably the sphincter of the

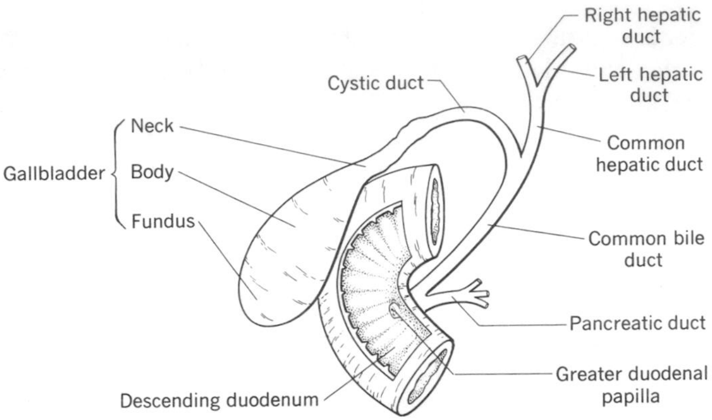

Figure 1 depicts the extrahepatic biliary passages in the typical arrangement.

common bile duct, which delay the emptying of stomach and gall bladder. The acute flare-ups or biliary colics found in our case as in many others are caused by impaction of stones in the neck of the gall bladder.

Name the various parts of the gall bladder that are involved in this case. They are the fundus, body, and neck of the gall bladder, with the neck opening into the cystic duct (Fig. 1).

Anatomy of biliary pain and rigidity

Typical for biliary colic is the appearance of sudden, sharp, severe pain that starts in the epigastric and umbilical regions and then becomes localized in the right hypochondriac area and radiates toward the inferior angle of the scapula and caudal to it.

How do you explain the location of pain in the right hypochondriac region and its typical radiation to the back, particularly to the scapular and infrascapular area? The pain in the right hypochondriac area is caused by direct inflammatory stimulation of the sensory nerve endings in the parietal peritoneum overlying the gall bladder. The pain in the scapular region is referred pain, which is common in diseases involving the viscera. For physiologic reasons pain arising in sensory nerve endings in the viscus, that is, the gall bladder, is referred to areas of the body surface that send sensory impulses to the same segment of the spinal cord that receives sensation from the affected organs.

Sensory fibers from the gall bladder run in plexuses along the biliary duct, closely intermingled with sympathetic efferent fibers. They pass through the celiac ganglion, the greater splanchnic nerve, sympathetic chain ganglia, and via white rami communicantes to spinal nerves and their dorsal roots and ganglia. Here their cell bodies are located. Central fibers from the ganglia terminate in the seventh to ninth thoracic cord segments. It is in the dermatomes derived from these cord segments that the radiating pain to the scapular and infrascapular area is localized.

Explain the muscular rigidity that is found over the diseased area. This rigidity is a state of involuntary contraction of the muscles of the anterior abdominal wall, particularly the rectus abdominis, which is a reflex response to stimulation of the nerve endings in the parietal peritoneum in the region of the gall bladder.

Topography of the abdomen

In our case history are used two different topographic terminologies that are frequently utilized in clinical descriptions. The simpler one divides the abdomen into four quadrants by a midsagittal and a horizontal plane laid through the umbilicus. A second more complex terminology introduces nine regions, outlined by two vertical and two horizontal planes.

What is the location of these planes and what are the names of the regions? The two vertical planes are erected from the midpoints of the inguinal ligaments, the upper horizontal plane is laid through the lowest point of the tenth costal cartilage, the lower horizontal plane passes through the level of the highest points of the iliac crest. The regions outlined are the right and left hypochondriac, the right and left lateral, the right and left inguinal, the epigastric, umbilical, and pubic.

Clinically important relations of the gall bladder

The abnormal findings in our case include the presence of dense adhesions to the organs in the neighborhood. Identify the organs that are in such intimate relationship to the gall bladder that not only adhesions may form between it and these viscera, but also rupture and discharge of pus and stones may occur from the gall bladder into these organs. They are the liver, the first part of the duodenum, the jejunum, and the transverse colon. Perforation may also occur into the peritoneal cavity or through the anterior abdominal wall. The greater omentum is frequently adherent to the gall bladder.

Is the gall bladder normally separated from the visceral surface of the liver by a layer of peritoneum? The gall bladder lodges in its own groove on the under surface of the liver, to the right of the quadrate lobe, with only connective tissue but no peritoneum intervening. The peritoneum which covers the visceral surface of the liver passes over the sides and inferior surface of the gall bladder without usually surrounding the latter or supplying it with a mesentery.

Although operations on the biliary tract are almost as common as surgery for inguinal hernia and appendicitis, complications in gall bladder surgery are far more frequent than in the other two operations. These complications are mainly due to lack of appreciation of anatomical variations that occur so frequently in the extrahepatic biliary system. A comprehensive knowledge of these anatomical deviations can prevent many complications. Cautious dissection will help in the identification of the important structures and will protect them from injury.

The first surgical step in cholecystectomy is an incision into the lesser omentum close to its free border. Define the lesser omentum and name the structures that are encountered between its two layers near its free (right) edge. The lesser omentum is a peritoneal duplicature derived from the ventral mesogastrium that connects the stomach and first part of the duodenum with the liver. Consequently its two continuous parts are named the hepatogastric and the hepatoduodenal ligaments. In cholecystectomy we are concerned with the latter. Between its two layers and close to its free margin lie three important structures: the common bile duct farthest to the right, the hepatic artery to the left of the common bile duct, and the portal vein between and posterior to them. (A justified mnemonic is: "*d*uctus-*d*exter, *p*ortal vein-*p*osterior.") Other structures surrounding this triad are nerve and lymph plexuses.

Anomalies of the cystic duct

It is the task of the surgeon first of all to identify the cystic duct, then doubly clamp, ligate, and divide it. With the liver and gall bladder retracted, the cystic duct, about 3 to 4 cm in length, runs posteriorly, caudally, and to the left, and joins the common hepatic duct to form with it the common bile duct (choledochus). Most important to the surgeon are variations in length and course of the cystic duct and the site of junction with the common hepatic duct (Fig. 2). If the cystic duct is unusually long, it may run in apposition to the common hepatic duct for a variable length of the latter's course, often attached to it by connective tissue. The cystic duct, instead of joining the common hepatic duct on its right side, may pass in front or behind the common duct uniting with it on its left side (Fig. 2). If the anomalies mentioned are not recognized, the common duct may be mistaken for the cystic duct and may be clamped, ligated, or even partially resected. Blind clamping or ligation of bleeding blood vessels may also lead to injuries or occlusion of the common duct.

The result of complete occlusion of the common duct is severe jaundice, which is fatal unless the patient is reoperated. Patency of the common duct must be reestablished or bile drainage otherwise instituted. Milder injuries to the common bile duct lead to drainage of bile into the subhepatic area and through the drain to the outside, which may or may not require surgical intervention. If large amounts of bile enter the free peritoneal cavity, bile peritonitis results and possibly death from shock.

Anomalies of the cystic artery

The recognition of vascular anomalies, particularly of the cystic artery, is of equal clinical importance. The typical arrangement to be described occurs in only two-thirds of all

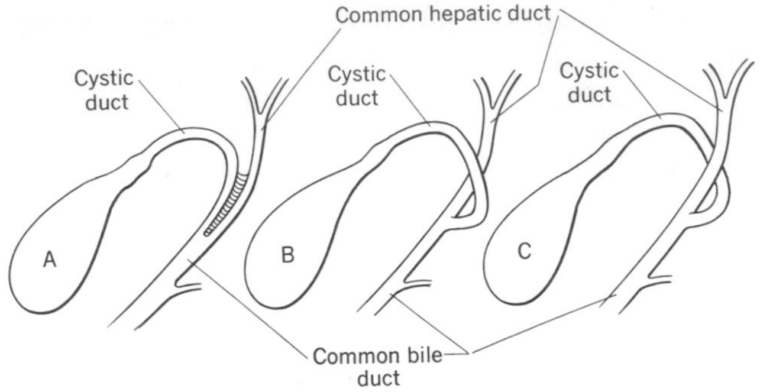

Figure 2A shows an unusually long cystic duct, attached to the common hepatic duct by connective tissue. Figure 2B shows the cystic duct joining the common hepatic duct on its left side by passing in front of it. Figure 2C shows the cystic duct joining the common hepatic duct on its left side by passing behind it.

cases. Here the cystic artery arises from the right hepatic artery to the right of the hepatic duct. After a course that is variable in length the artery divides into a superficial and a deep branch, one going to the peritoneal, the other to the attached surface of the gall bladder. The cystic artery may also arise from the hepatic artery proper at the site of its bifurcation or before it divides into the right and left branch. Other rarer origins of the cystic artery are from a hepatic artery that is a branch of the superior mesenteric artery. Finally there may be accessory cystic branches from any of the previously mentioned arteries.

If the surgeon is unfamiliar with the possible multiplicity of the cystic artery or its abnormal course, profuse unexpected hemorrhage may result, which can be temporarily controlled by compressing the hepatic artery between index finger and thumb within the layers of the lesser omentum. If the right hepatic artery is mistaken for the cystic artery, and if it is ligated instead of the cystic artery, necrosis of the liver occurs, resulting in serious consequences and possibly death. Significant postoperative hemorrhage from injury to abnormal blood vessels is a grave complication that requires immediate reoperation. It is best avoided by carefully identifying all blood vessels at the time of cholecystectomy, being always aware of the possibility of aberrant blood vessels.

23 "Dropped" Stomach

A 32-year-old unmarried schoolteacher is referred by her physician to the outpatient department with the diagnosis of gastroptosis ("dropped" stomach) and dyspepsia. The patient complains of frequent nausea, heartburn, occasional vomiting, and a sense of fullness and abdominal discomfort soon after intake of food. The attacks of vomiting occur when she is upset in her work as a teacher.

In the last few months, after the death of her mother with whom she lived, her symptoms have become increasingly severe. She now complains also of frequent headaches, fatigue upon slight exertion, insomnia, and loss of appetite.

EXAMINATION

The patient appears frail, underdeveloped, and undernourished. The epigastrium is slightly sensitive on palpation, but there are no other abnormalities. The radiologic examination of the gastrointestinal tract shows the stomach lacking in tonus; the stomach is quite long, sagging down into the lesesr pelvis with the lowest point of the greater curvature three fingerbreadths above the symphysis pubis. The pylorus is at the level of the fifth lumbar vertebra to the left of the midline (Fig. 1). There are no signs of organic changes in the stomach or duodenum. The stomach empties fairly normally, being free of contrast medium after four and a half hours. On radiographic examination of the gall bladder, the gall bladder

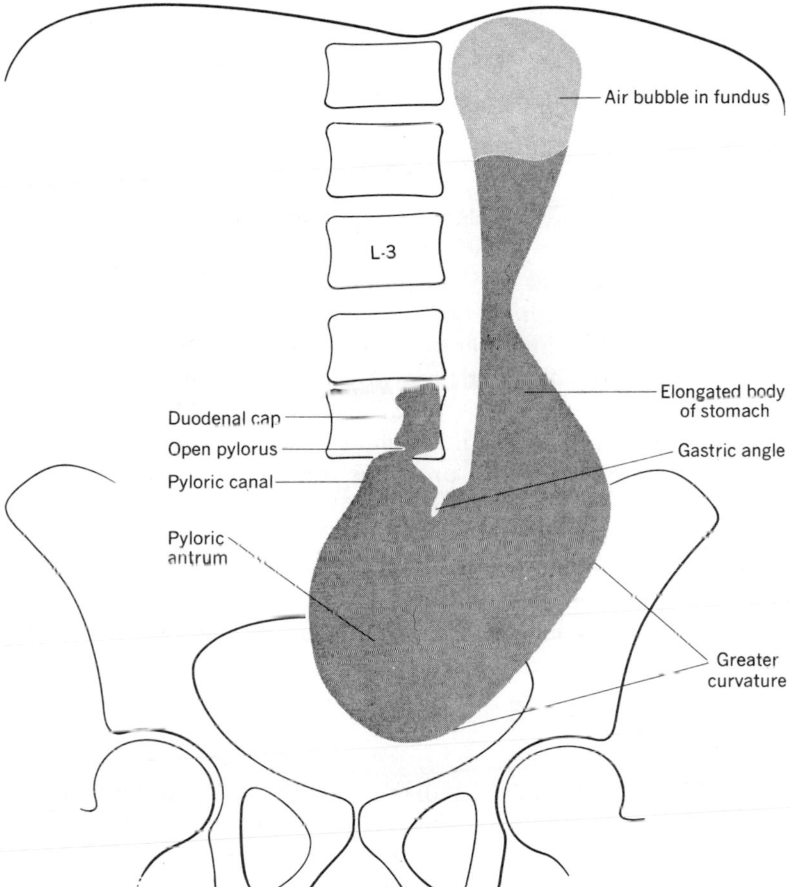

Figure 1 shows elongated stomach of low tonus with the lowest point of the greater curvature three fingerbreadths above the symphysis pubis. The pylorus is at the level of the fifth lumbar vertebra to the left of the midline. This finding is consistent with normal function.

appears elongated and low in position, but otherwise normal. There are therefore no signs of organic abnormalities in the upper gastrointestinal tract.

DIAGNOSIS

Stomach distress on an emotional, non-organic basis.

THERAPY AND FURTHER COURSE

During follow-up, the patient is seen on numerous occasions by a psychiatrically oriented physician. In these interviews she reveals that she feels insufficient for her tasks, particularly since the death of her mother on whom she relied heavily. She appears hypersensitive to frustrations and reacts to them emotionally and with the previously described gastric symptoms.

With the physician assuming a sympathetic and supportive attitude toward her problems, the patient's health gradually improves. She gains more confidence in herself, and her gastric symptoms are greatly alleviated. Under dietary supervision, mild sedation, and symptomatic medical treatment—and with continuance of occasional psychotherapeutic interviews—the patient has gained fifteen pounds and finds her mild gastric discomfort quite tolerable.

DISCUSSION

The original clinical diagnosis by her local physician was gastroptosis, which refers to descent and sagging of the stomach, this condition supposedly being responsible for her clinical symptoms. The term implies a "standard" or "normal" position of the stomach from which the patient's organ deviates in a caudal direction.

Position of the stomach in the cadaver and in the living

What is the "normal" position of the stomach? The formulation of the question in this manner, although frequently posed in the clinical and anatomical literature, is incorrect and unacceptable. The concept of a "standard" or "normal" gastric position is based on data collected at the turn of the century by the British anatomist Addison. He divided the abdominal region into small squares and allotted to the viscera fixed places in this scheme. The opinion prevailed that each organ, thoracic, abdominal, or pelvic, has its definite shape and position, a knowledge of which was necessary to recognize deviations. The corollary of this theory was the assumption that deviation from this standard position, particularly in a caudal direction, results in clinical symptoms. The descent or sagging of a viscus was called "ptosis," and the literature of the past is replete with descriptions and case histories of gastroptosis, coloptosis, and generalized enteroptosis. Surgical procedures were devised which aimed at anchoring organs in their "allotted" location. As recently as a few years ago the surgical literature mentioned various techniques of surgical "gastropexy," which meant the fixation of a "dropped" stomach in a higher position by suturing it to the abdominal wall or other structures.

Addison's work consisted of a statistical evaluation of variations in the topography of abdominal organs in the cadaver. What factors make the position of an organ in a cadaver a very unreliable index of its location in the living? What is the state of the smooth and striated musculature in the dead body? What are the postmortem pressure conditions in the abdomen? The smooth and striated musculature, which includes the diaphragm, is either completely relaxed or abnormally rigid due to rigor mortis. The thorax is in a state of maximal expiration with collapse of the lung and elevation of the diaphragm. Embalming and dissecting procedures change the pressure conditions in the thoracic and abdominal cavities and within the vasculature. The elasticity of connective tissue is lost and the fat is solidified.

Thus, the study of visceral topographic anatomy in the dissecting room is of very limited value in the assessment of visceral shape and position in the living. Yet even the modern anatomical and clinical literature frequently ignores the available evidence of this discrepancy. Thus, a recent anatomical work analyzes and illustrates topographic findings on abdominal viscera as encountered after the abdomen of embalmed cadavers has been opened.

Returning to the living, list the physiologic variables that lead to alterations in the position of the stomach and other abdominal viscera. Body posture and respiratory phase are responsible for a wide range of shape and position of the abdominal viscera. The stomach descends in the upright position and with the descent of the diaphragm, that is, in inspiration. If you were to demonstrate on two consecutive X-ray films extremes of variation in gastric position, how would you manipulate the variables of respiration and body position? One film would be taken in inspiration and in upright position and the other in expiration and supine position.

What other striated muscles, in addition to the diaphragm, affect gastric position? The state of contraction of the muscles of the anterior abdominal wall has the greatest influence on the position of the stomach. This can easily be demonstrated under the fluoroscope by letting the subject retract his abdomen or by causing sudden contractions of the anterior abdominal wall by making the subject laugh. Needless to say that the degree of filling of the stomach will alter its position—although not to the extent that classical anatomists assumed—and sc does the state of filling and size of organs in the neighborhood, such as the colon and spleen.

Tonus of the stomach

What is meant by the term "tone" or "tonus" of the stomach, and how does it affect gastric location? Tonus, in contrast to peristalsis, refers to the continuous state of contraction of the smooth musculature of the stomach. In our patient we find considerable loss of tone, in other words, a relaxation of the gastric wall, resulting in a caudally directed outpouching, especially of the greater curvature.

What nerve structures govern the tonus of the smooth musculature of the stomach? The latter is mainly under control of the intrinsic myenteric plexus in the wall of the organ but is also influenced by its extrinsic innervation, the vagus and sympathetic. What are the results of vagal or sympathetic stimulation on the tonus of the stomach? They are not clear-cut, but depend on the degree of tonus at the time of stimulation as well as on the frequency and strength of the stimulus. In general the vagus increases the tonus of the organ while the sympathetic is inhibitory to the stomach wall. There is evidence of cortical and subcortical control of gastric tonus. Centers in the cortex most likely act upon the hypothalamus, which in turn affects the vagal and sympathetic outflow. Acute emotional upsets result in increased activity of the thoracolumbar division of the autonomic nervous system and of the adrenal medulla and are therefore generally accompanied by a decrease in tonus of the gastric wall and a sagging of the stomach. Thus we understand that the temporary emotional disturbance of our patient enhanced the descent of her stomach.

How do the autonomic components of the nervous system reach the stomach? The stomach is supplied from the celiac plexus via postganglionic sympathetic nerve fibers which follow the gastric arteries. Preganglionic vagal fibers reach the organ by direct gastric branches from the two vagal trunks or through the celiac plexus which receives a parasympathetic contribution. Most of the preganglionic vagal fibers synapse in the intrinsic autonomic plexuses of the organ.

Stomach and constitutional type

If physiologic variables such as body posture, respiratory phase, and state of filling of the stomach and adjacent viscera are standardized and emotional upsets are excluded, is there conformity in the site of the organ? Studies on groups of people, even of the same age, have shown that gastric position correlates to a certain extent with body build. Persons with frail and slender physique, such as our patient, generally show a lower diaphragm and a lack of tonus of the skeletal musculature with sagging of the anterior abdominal wall and to a certain extent of the pelvic support of the viscera. This, combined with the spaciousness of the pelvis and the scarcity of abdominal fat, results in a low position of the viscera, including the stomach. On the other hand, in the heavy-set stocky individual with a high diaphragm and roomy upper abdomen the viscera generally are in a more cranial position.

Transpyloric plane and stomach bed

Two conventional anatomical terms referring to the stomach, the so-called transpyloric plane and the stomach bed, require further elucidation. What is your definition of the transpyloric plane which was introduced by Addison and which by its name seems to refer to the site of the pylorus? The transpyloric plane is a horizontal plane midway between the suprasternal notch and the pubic symphysis. It is supposed to pass through the disk between the first and the second lumbar vertebra. In what position in the living is the pylorus most apt to lie in or near this plane? In an X-ray anatomical study it was shown that, with the subject supine, the pylorus of the empty stomach was in the transpyloric plane in approximately 20 per cent of all cases; in another approximately 15 per cent it was cranial to the transpyloric plane. But even in this position where the stomach is most elevated, the pylorus was caudal to the transpyloric plane in more than 60 per cent of all cases. For the erect male it was found that in no case did the pylorus lie in the transpyloric plane, but always caudal to it. Thus, for the living, particularly in the anatomical, that is, upright position, the term is a misnomer.

What is the definition of the stomach bed? It refers to the structures to which the posterior surface of the stomach is related in the supine position. What are these structures? They are from cranial to caudal, the diaphragm, the left suprarenal gland, a small part of the left kidney, the splenic artery along the upper border of the pancreas, the body of the pancreas, the spleen to the left of kidney and pancreas, and the transverse mesocolon descending from the pancreas. All these structures are separated from the stomach by the omental bursa. The spleen lies at the left extremity of the bursa, connected to the stomach by the gastrosplenic ligament. In the upright position the relationships of the stomach change greatly. The organ descends and rests essentially on the transverse mesocolon and adjacent intestines, which in turn are supported by the anterior abdominal wall and the pelvic organs.

What is the most fixed part of the organ? The cardia changes least in position with physiologic alterations. By contrast the pylorus is quite mobile, being suspended from the liver by the mesentery-like lesser omentum. The pylorus not only moves craniocaudally as has been pointed out, but also from right to left of the midline.

Where does the pylorus lie in our patient? In the upright position it is at the level of the fifth lumbar vertebra to the left of the midline (Fig. 1). The following well-worded quotation sums up this discussion on the stomach bed: "The stomach-bed, once given the rigidity of an ancient four-poster, now has become the malleable bed of a flowing river on which floats the visceral fleet" (O'Rahilly).

In conclusion it should be stated that normal function of the abdominal viscera does not depend on their position; that a stomach or transverse colon that has descended into the pelvis functions just as well as one that lies higher in the abdomen. There is, therefore, no justification for the clinical diagnosis of gastroptosis or coloptosis.

There is, however, one organ whose low position might cause clinical symptoms. What is this organ? Nephroptosis generally has been accepted as a clinical entity. Recently considerable doubt has arisen as to the validity of this concept for many cases. Low position of the kidney should be considered as a relatively normal finding. Only if one can demonstrate definite signs of obstruction of the pelvis of the kidney or urinary stasis by kinking of the ureter, is he justified in regarding the downward displacement of the kidney as a pathological condition.

24 Perforated Ulcer of the Stomach

A 36-year-old bookkeeper was well until two years ago when he suffered periodic attacks of nausea, heartburn, and epigastric pain. During these periods the pain became worse when the stomach was empty and was relieved by food and antacids. The present illness started acutely soon after a heavy lunch when suddenly, while reaching over to a desk in his office, he experienced agonizing pain in his abdomen. A physician was called immediately and he transferred the patient to a hospital by ambulance.

EXAMINATION

On arrival at the hospital the pain was still excruciating and sharp, knife-like in character. It was located in the epigastrium and was constant, but from time to time increasing in intensity. The patient appeared prostrated. His face had an anxious expression and his forehead was covered with cold sweat. His breathing was rapid and shallow, and the abdominal wall did not seem to participate in respiratory movements. The temperature was normal, the pulse rate was only slightly elevated, and the blood pressure was normal. There was a board-like rigidity of the abdomen, most marked in the epigastric area and left hypochondriac region and somewhat less pronounced in the umbilical region. Abdominal tenderness on palpation was most marked in the epigastrium.

DIAGNOSIS

On the basis of the past history, which made the presence of a gastric or duodenal ulcer likely, the diagnosis of acute perforation of the ulcer was made and the patient was sent to the operating room. During the period the patient was prepared for surgery, the pain seemed to decrease slightly and there was some general improvement.

THERAPY

On opening of the abdomen under spinal anesthesia, the general peritoneal cavity showed the presence of moderate amounts of turbid fluid and some food particles, which were removed by suction. No sign of a ruptured ulcer on the duodenum or anterior wall of the stomach was demonstrable however. In view of the clinical findings and the presence of fluid and food in the peritoneal cavity, perforation of an ulcer on the posterior wall into the omental bursa (lesser sac) was assumed and the omental bursa opened by an incision through the gastrocolic ligament, avoiding the blood vessels along the greater curvature of the stomach. In the bursa a considerable amount of gastric secretion and food was found which was removed by suction. The stomach was turned upward for adequate exposure and a perforated ulcer, one-half cm. in diameter was visualized, 2 cm. from the lesser curvature on the posterior aspect of the body of the stomach (Fig. 1). The ulcer was excised, and frozen sections of the ulcerous area showed it to be nonmalignant. In the absence of cancer the defect in the stomach was closed.

FURTHER COURSE

The patient had a fairly stormy convalescence with spiking temperatures. The postoperative care included constant gastric suction through a stomach tube, intravenous fluids, and antibiotics. The patient gradually improved and was put on a strict ulcer diet. Three weeks after operation, being greatly

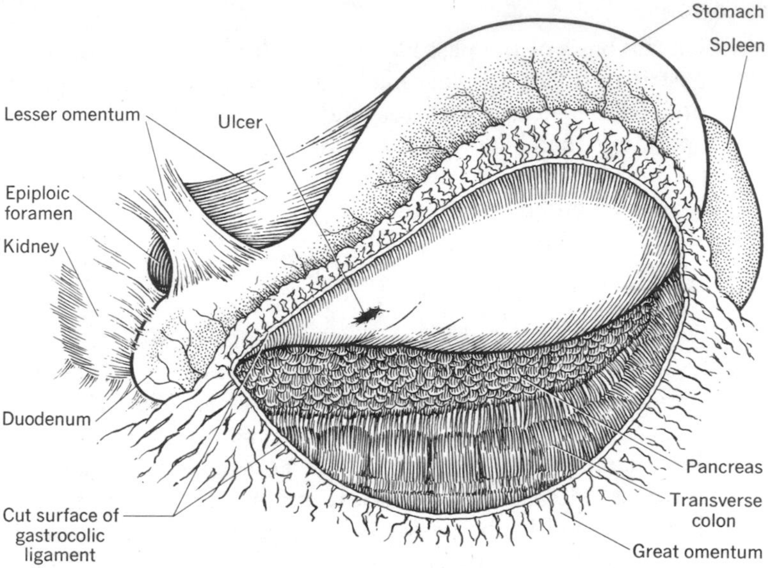

Figure 1—The omental bursa has been opened by an incision through the gastrocolic ligament. The stomach has been turned up and the perforated ulcer is shown on the posterior aspect of the body of the stomach, fairly close to the lesser curvature.

improved, he was discharged and was continued on his diet. Three months after operation he was reported recovered and working.

DISCUSSION

The outstanding symptoms in this patient are abdominal tenderness, which is abnormal sensitiveness to touch, and the excruciating pain. The latter made immediate intervention necessary.

Anatomy of ulcer pain

In dealing with the anatomy of the various modalities of pain present in this case, we have to separate the chronic ulcer pain that the patient complained of in his history, and which is often described as gnawing and ill-defined in location, from the sharp, stabbing pain after the perforation had taken place. The former, often identified as visceral, is mediated through afferent fibers that accompany the sympathetic efferent fibers from the wall of the stomach through the celiac ganglia, greater splanchnic nerves, sympathetic chain ganglia, white rami communicantes, spinal nerves, then by way of posterior roots to spinal ganglia. Here their cell bodies are located. Central fibers from these ganglion cells continue into the spinal cord. Pain of this type, elicited in the stomach by the ulcer, is generally referred to the epigastric region. By contrast, the sharp, knife-like pain after perforation is due to peritoneal irritation by the gastric secretion and contents. It is mediated by somatic sensory fibers of the body wall which supply the parietal peritoneum. Remember that the parietal peritoneum, as well as the skin, in the area of the umbilicus is supplied by the tenth intercostal nerve. Thus the sharp pain, which is fairly well localized in the epigastric region starting just below the xiphoid process, would point to involvement of the sixth to the ninth intercostal nerves. Does the vagus conduct sensory impulses from the stomach including pain? It seems to mediate mainly those sensory impulses concerned with gastric reflexes, but it is generally assumed not to transmit pain from the stomach.

What is the cause of the rigidity of the abdominal wall and the costal character of the patient's respiration? The rigidity is due to contraction of the muscular wall and is a reflex response of the abdominal muscles to abnormal stimuli arising from the involved area. The costal type of breathing with avoidance of abdominal respiratory excursions can be explained as a protective mechanism shielding the abdominal wall and parietal peritoneum from painful movements.

Surgical anatomy of the omental bursa

The perforation in this case involves the omental bursa into which the gastric secretions and food have spilled through the

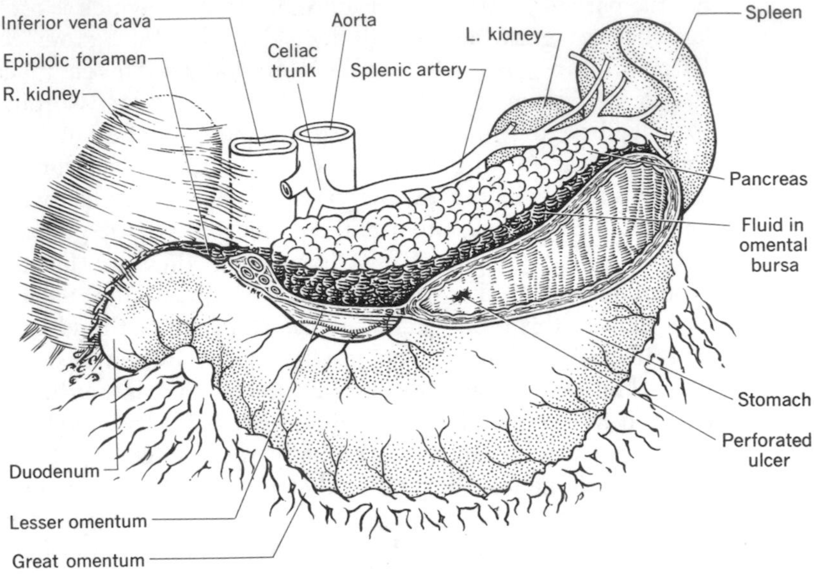

Figure 2—Shows a cross section through the stomach above the level of the perforated ulcer. Notice the collection of fluid in the omental bursa and its communication with the general peritoneal cavity through the epiploic foramen. Also notice the relation of the pancreas and splenic artery to the posterior wall of the stomach, separated from it only by the omental bursa.

opening of the perforated ulcer (Fig. 2). How do you explain the presence of extraneous material in the general peritoneal cavity? Does the peritoneal cavity communicate with the omental bursa? Locate the epiploic foramen which is the opening of the bursa into the peritoneal cavity and give its boundaries. The foramen is bounded anteriorly by the free (right) border of the lesser omentum, containing the common bile duct, the hepatic artery, and the portal vein; posteriorly by the inferior vena cava; superiorly by the caudate lobe of the liver; and inferiorly by the first part of the duodenum (Fig. 2). What aspect of the stomach bounds the bursa anteriorly? Perforating lesions of what portion of the stomach would be most apt to involve the bursa? Into what space do ulcers of the anterior wall of the stomach perforate? Is the lesser omentum part of the anterior wall of the bursa? The lesser omentum and the posterior wall of the stomach form the important anterior boundaries of the main part of the omental bursa. Thus while ulcers of the anterior wall of the stomach are apt to perforate into the free peritoneal cavity (greater sac), ulcers of the posterior wall may rupture into the omental bursa (lesser sac), as in our case.

Recesses of the omental bursa

What is meant by the terms "superior and inferior recesses" of the omental bursa? What lobe of the liver, covered by peritoneum, forms part of the boundary of the bursa? How do you explain variations in the caudal extent of the inferior recess? If this recess extended into the greater omentum, between which layers of the omentum would it be located? Would this variable extension of the inferior recess be anterior or posterior to the transverse colon? The superior recess extends behind the liver, with the caudate lobe protruding into it from above. The inferior recess between the inner two layers of the greater omentum is of variable extent caudally, depending on the degree of fusion of these layers. Usually it reaches only as far as the transverse colon, but would extend anterior to it, if the layers of the greater omentum remained unfused.

Pancreas and the omental bursa

Normally the space of the bursa is only potential, so that the posterior wall of the stomach is in contact with the anterior aspect of the pancreas, separated only by two layers of peritoneum. What are these? They are the serosal covering of the posterior wall of the stomach and the peritoneum lining the posterior wall of the bursa in front of the pancreas. Consequently which organ is most apt to be invaded if an ulcer on the posterior wall of the stomach slowly perforates through the gastric wall? Actually penetration into the pancreas from posterior gastric ulcer, with fixation of the stomach to the anterior aspect of the pancreas and walling off of this perforation by peritoneal adhesions, is more common than the massive acute perforation described in this case. What major branch of the celiac trunk would be subject to erosion and possible fatal hemorrhage if this slow perforation and fixation were directed along the upper margin of the pancreas? The splenic artery would be involved.

Surgical access to the bursa

How was the omental bursa (lesser sac) opened in this case? Strictly speaking, the term "gastrocolic ligament" denotes that portion of the greater omentum which extends from the greater curvature of the stomach to the transverse colon and implies that the lower part of the omental bursa is obliterated. If it were patent, then the same surgical result would be obtained by going through the anterior two layers of the greater omentum. What vessels in the uppermost portion of this peritoneal duplicature have to be avoided in this surgical approach? The right and left gastroepiploic arteries form an anastomotic arch caudal to the greater curvature of the stomach. Remember that the term "epiploic" in the name of these vessels refers to the greater omentum.

What further accesses to the lesser sac could be utilized in addition to the narrow pathway through the epiploic foramen and the inadvisable approach through the lesser omentum? Entrance could also be obtained by going from below through the transverse mesocolon although at the risk of injuring the artery to this part of the colon. Name and locate this artery and give its origin. The middle colic artery, a large branch of the superior mesenteric artery, runs between the layers of the transverse mesocolon. British surgeons have occasionally recommended access to the omental bursa through the gastrolienal ligament. Locate it. What vessels would be endangered in this approach? The surgeon has to guard against injury to the short gastric and left gastroepiploic vessels which run within the gastrolienal ligament.

25 Arteriomesenteric Occlusion of Duodenum

A 33-year-old medical secretary comes to the physician's office complaining of nausea and vomiting of bile-stained food, with sensations of bloating, belching, discomfort, and pain in the upper abdomen. These symptoms come on approximately one to two hours after meals. Following a respiratory infection she suffered a marked weight loss amounting to twenty-five pounds during the last six months. Since then her symptoms have gradually worsened.

On inquiry she states that since adolescence she has had alternating periods of well-being and abdominal discomfort accompanied by vomiting. Since the recent aggravation of her symptoms, she has felt very fatigued and has lost her appetite. She further states that when she has these attacks of pain and vomiting she can obtain relief by lying on her side or in the knee-chest position.

EXAMINATION

On physical examination we find a rather apprehensive patient of asthenic habitus. The latter is particularly conspicuous since she shows evidence of recent marked weight loss. She has very flaccid abdominal walls and her liver, kidneys, and spleen can be palpated easily. As is common in asthenic individuals, she has a marked lumbar lordosis. The epigastrium is rather tender, but otherwise no signs of acute intestinal illness, such as rigidity of the abdominal wall or indications of intestinal obstruction, can be elicited. The patient is advised to seek admittance to the hospital for further studies.

In the hospital a full-blown attack is observed, which came on after a fairly large meal with a meat course and dessert. She was stricken with nausea and fairly severe cramping pain in the right upper abdominal quadrant. She vomited bile-stained food which she had eaten recently. The vomiting relieved her pain. Before the attack subsided, the examining physician noted that the patient displayed tenderness and visible peristalsis in the right upper abdominal region.

Radiographic study of the upright patient under the fluoroscope with a radiopaque meal shows rapid emptying of the stomach, which permits exclusion of pyloric stenosis. The first three portions of the duodenum fill rapidly and are considerably dilated. Under active peristalsis the duodenum finally empties part of the barium into its fourth portion, but there is marked indentation of the barium filling at the site of transition of the third and fourth portions of the duodenum to the right of the third and fourth lumbar vertebra. This corresponds to the cutoff point at the time of the beginning of filling of the duodenum. X-ray examination six hours after the barium meal shows a marked and abnormal residue of barium in the duodenum.

DIAGNOSIS

Chronic type of arteriomesenteric occlusion of the duodenum.

FURTHER COURSE AND THERAPY

The patient is put on a strict diet with small caloric liquid feedings every two hours. She is advised to assume alternatingly the prone, right and left lateral, and knee-chest positions, the latter particularly after meals. Since she prefers to sleep in the supine position during the night, the foot of the bed is elevated during this period. Gradually her meals are increased in frequency and solids are added. She is allowed to get up intermittently, first for short periods. The time out of bed is increased gradually. She is also given exercises to strengthen her abdominal muscles. During the next two weeks, she gains 10 pounds and her attacks of pain become less frequent. She is discharged from the hospital with a recommendation to assume the supine or knee-chest position after each meal. She is also given an abdominal binder for support and told to exercise her abdominal muscles. She continues her weight gain and shows overall improvement in her general well-being, accompanied by decreased frequency of abdominal attacks. She is allowed, therefore, to return to work. Six months later she has regained her normal weight and she feels comfortable. Her attacks occur quite infrequently, not more than once or twice a month. She is advised to be careful about her diet by avoiding coarse or stringy foods and to continue her muscle-strengthening exercises.

DISCUSSION

Obstruction of the third portion of the duodenum as a clinical entity is an interesting phenomenon. Enthusiasm for this diagnosis has waxed and waned since the disease was first defined in the middle of the last century. There are still authors who deny the occurrence of such an entity, but the majority of clinicians are now convinced of its existence, particularly when confirmed by radiographic evidence. What are the underlying facts? Anatomists and pathologists have known for a long time that the postmortem casts of the duodenum frequently show an imprint of the superior mesenteric vessels on the anterior wall of the third part of the duodenum. The equivalent of this imprint has been demonstrated *in vivo* by radiologic means as a filling defect in the same location.

Underlying anatomy of the condition

Define the third part of the duodenum. What is its relation to adjacent structures, particularly the parietal peritoneum, transverse colon, mesocolon, pancreas, aorta, and superior mesenteric vessels? In the early part of his training the medical student, in his dissection, and the surgeon, at the operating table, frequently have difficulty identifying this portion of the duodenum since it lies entirely retroperitoneal and is crossed by the mesentery from which the loops of the small intestine are suspended. It is also overlain by the transverse mesocolon and transverse colon. The latter structures have to be lifted cranially and the mesentery of the small intestine turned to the left to expose the parietal peritoneum of the posterior abdominal wall that covers the third part of the duodenum. It then can be palpated to the right of the mesenteric root. This part of the duodenum, which is also often called the inferior or horizontal portion, is about three inches in length. It begins at the inferior duodenal flexure as the continuation of the descending portion and generally crosses the third lumbar vertebra. At its left extremity it becomes the fourth or ascending portion which terminates as the duodenojejunal flexure (Fig. 1 and 2).

As stated previously, the third part of the duodenum is covered ventrally by the parietal peritoneum except for a small area where the superior mesenteric vessels cross it at the site of transition of the third into the fourth part of the duodenum to enter the mesenteric root. It is separated from the spinal column by the inferior vena cava to the right of the column and the abdominal aorta in front of the column. The transverse mesocolon, with the transverse colon suspended from it, crosses cranial to the third part of the duodenum by passing over the second or descending portion of the duodenum. The transverse mesocolon divides the duodenum into supra- and infracolic portions. The pancreas is likewise cranial to the third part of the duodenum.

Superior mesenteric artery and vein

The superior mesenteric artery is given off the front of the aorta as the second of the unpaired visceral arteries (the celiac trunk being the first), generally at the level of the lower portion of the first lumbar vertebra and therefore cranial to the third part of the duodenum. The artery is accompanied by its vein as it passes over the third part of the duodenum to enter the

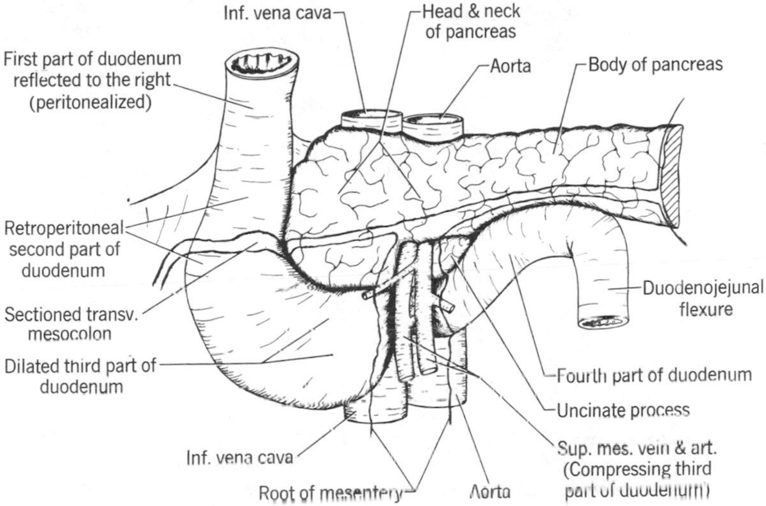

Figure 1—Front view of duodenum in a case of arteriomesenteric occlusion of third portion of duodenum. Notice the prestenotic dilatation of the duodenum and compression of its third portion by root of mesentery and superior mesenteric vessels. Observe that the superior mesenteric artery arises from the aorta posterior to the neck of the pancreas but crosses in front of the uncinate process. The crossing of the root of the transverse mesocolon over the second portion of the duodenum and the anterior surface of the pancreas is also shown.

mesentery and to supply the small and large intestines from the distal duodenum to the left colic flexure. The superior mesenteric vein drains the same area of intestine and courses to the right of the artery (Figs. 1 and 2). Their relationship to each other is easy to remember if one keeps in mind that the artery arises from the aorta in the midsagittal plane while the vein drains into the portal vein in its course towards the liver which is essentially a right-sided organ.

What is the relation of the superior mesenteric artery to the pancreas? It arises from the aorta behind the neck of the pancreas but crosses in front of the uncinate process of the pancreas. In its course, the artery is surrounded by the superior

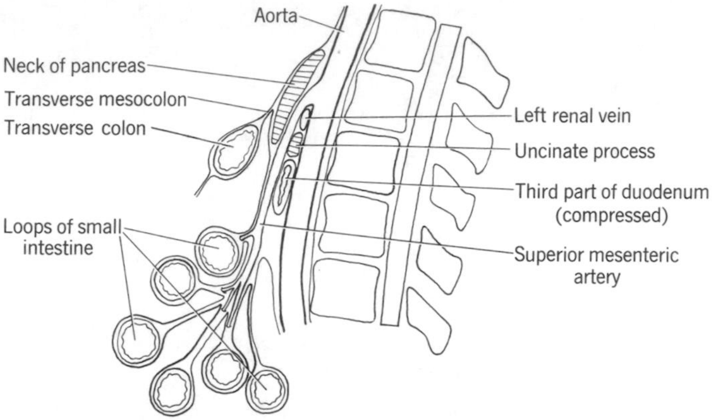

Figure 2—Midsagittal section showing superior mesenteric artery stretched over the third portion of the duodenum and left renal vein by low-lying loops of small intestine in case of severe loss of weight and depletion of mesenteric fat. Notice compression of third portion of duodenum. The normal relationship of the artery behind the neck but in front of the uncinate process of the pancreas is also shown.

mesenteric nerve plexus. Since the artery runs posterior to the neck of the pancreas it is, of course, also posterior to the transverse mesocolon which arises from the anterior surface of the pancreas. It is worthwhile to keep in mind that, while the origin of the superior mesenteric artery is cranial to the third portion of the duodenum, the origin of the inferior mesenteric artery is caudal to this part of the duodenum. It is also easy to remember that the superior and inferior mesenteric veins, which accompany the two mesenteric arteries, both lie to the outside of the arteries, i.e. closer to the lateral abdominal wall than the arteries.

The changing position of the duodenum

Since the duodenum, with the exception of its first portion, is a retroperitoneal structure, its position is less variable than organs having a mesentery. Nevertheless, it is surprising to observe that the duodenum is relatively mobile *in vivo.* Its location varies with body posture being lowest in the upright and highest in the prone position. It also changes with the degree of its filling and the state of contraction of the anterior abdominal wall. It descends with age. Thus, the level of the third lumbar vertebra or of the disk caudal to it, represents only a mean as a landmark for locating the third portion of the duodenum, with the range extending from L2 to L5.

Embryological explanation of the retroperitoneal and retrovascular position of the third part of the duodenum

How do you explain on an embryological basis the retroperitoneal position of the major part of the duodenum and the retrovascular location of the third portion of this viscus in relation to the superior mesenteric vessels? During embryonic development the intestinal tube forms an anteriorly convex loop in the midsagittal plane and is suspended from the dorsal wall of the abdomen by a mesentery. The tube rapidly increases in length and, adjusting to the available space, undergoes a counterclockwise rotation by 270° as viewed from the front, with the superior mesenteric artery acting as the axis of rotation. As the distal part of the intestinal loop turns over the proximal portion, the superior mesenteric artery comes to lie in front of the third part of the duodenum but posterior to the transverse colon. At a later stage the duodenum, together with certain other portions of the intestinal tract, loses its mesentery by peritoneal fusion and except for its first portion, becomes fixed to the posterior abdominal wall in a retroperitoneal position.

Pathogenesis of arteriomesenteric occlusion of the duodenum

The cardinal point of this discussion is, of course, the pathogenesis (i.e. mode of origin and development) of the clinical entity exemplified by our patient. While normally the superior mesenteric vessels pass gently over the third part of the duodenum, in our case we have to visualize the transverse duodenum as being markedly compressed, as in a vise, between the aorta and/or lordotic vertebral column posteriorly and the tautened mesenteric vessels anteriorly. This happens if, due to severe weight loss in an asthenic patient with insufficient abdominal muscular support, the intestines drop caudally to an undue degree. Thus, marked traction is exerted on the superior mesenteric vessels at the site of the mesenteric root. This can lead to acute or intermittent chronic obstruction of the duodenum at this level.

Asthenic habitus

What is meant by the term "asthenic habitus," so well demonstrated by our patient? The asthenic habitus represents one extreme of a continuous spectrum which extends from the short, stout, and stocky individual with well-developed musculature and heavy bony framework, to a body type characterized by tall, frail, and slender stature with a delicate skeleton, weak and underdeveloped musculature, and a low gastrointestinal tract reaching down into the pelvis. Other terms beside "asthenic" used for this body type are ectomorphic and linear. Such a body build is perfectly consistent with normal health and body function, as has been discussed in case study #23.

Explanation of symptoms

How do you explain the symptoms of the patient in the acute stages of her illness? What is the reason for the intermittent occurrence of her attacks with free intervals in between? From her history we learn that she has had acute periods of illness characterized by nausea, vomiting, belching, and pain in the right upper abdomen since adolescence. This is consistent with intermittent compression of the third part of the duodenum as the cause of the described symptoms. Vomiting temporarily relieves the overloading of stomach and duodenum proximal to the site of the compression. The free intervals, which may vary in length, can be explained by the force of peristalsis overcoming the obstruction and propelling the contents into the jejunum. The X-ray examination in our patient reveals, in addition to the dilatation of the duodenum proximal to the obstruction, increased peristalsis leading to emptying of the duodenum through the duodenojejunal flexure. Records of other cases also show hypertrophy of the duodenal musculature with dilatation proximal to the obstruction. It is understandable that incomplete constriction can become complete with exhaustion of the propelling muscular force. We then face an acute, life-threatening clinical picture that requires immediate surgery.

The recent aggravation of all symptoms in our patient is due to severe loss of weight and increased flaccidity of her abdominal musculature. The weight loss has resulted in diminution of the fat cushion in the mesenteric root which so far had protected the duodenum from complete and lasting compression. The accompanying loss of fat in the pelvis, greater omentum, and retroperitoneal structures, and the weakening of her abdominal musculature, has led to further sagging of the intestines into the pelvis and an increase of the drag on the mesenteric vessels. This further decreases the acute angle between aorta and superior mesenteric artery, a process that has been compared with the action of a nutcracker clamping down on the third part of the duodenum.

Clinicians and radiologists have reported that manual pressure on the lower abdomen in a cephalic direction with the patient in the supine position will relieve the retention by lifting the intestine out of the true pelvis. Pathologists have obtained similar results at autopsy by raising the viscera after opening of the peritoneal cavity, and have observed the passage of liquid contents or air beyond the point of obstruction after this maneuver.

What other factors may contribute to arteriomesenteric occlusion by tightening the vise on the inferior part of the duodenum? The patient's swayback or accentuated lumbar lordosis, which frequently accompanies the asthenic habitus particularly in the female, in combination with the defective abdominal musculature, increases the constriction.

Contributing developmental abnormalities

What faults in the development of the intestinal tract and its peritoneal relations can accentuate the tendency to obstruct the duodenum? A mobile cecum and an ascending colon suspended by a mesentery will exert traction on their supply arteries, thus increasing the pull on the superior mesenteric artery and the degree of compression of the duodenum. Occasionally a rigid arteriosclerotic superior mesenteric artery is thought to be a contributing factor.

Duodenal arterial supply from the superior mesenteric artery

It has been mentioned previously that the superior mesenteric artery contributes to the blood supply of the duodenum. Which arteries does it use? At the level of the pancreatic notch it gives off the inferior pancreaticoduodenal artery which then divides into two branches, an anterior and a posterior inferior pancreaticoduodenal artery. These form arcades between the pancreas and the descending part of the duodenum by communicating with the superior pancreaticoduodenal arteries from the gastroduodenal artery. They thus establish an important anastomosis between the celiac and superior mesenteric arteries.

Left renal vein exposed to compression

Is there another important blood vessel located in the angle between the aorta and superior mesenteric artery which may likewise be compressed by the pull of the superior mesenteric vessels? The left renal vein in its course toward the inferior vena cava crosses the aorta deep to the origin of the superior mesenteric artery above the third part of the duodenum. It has been asserted that increased acuteness in the previously mentioned angle may cause compression of this renal vein and circulatory changes in the left kidney, sometimes resulting in albuminuria (Fig. 2).

Surgery for treatment of arterio-mesenteric occlusion of the duodenum

Fortunately for the patient, her complaints were relieved by conservative medical management, but there remains a small percentage of cases which require surgery due to the severity and life-threatening character of their symptoms. The surgical treatment of duodenal obstruction consists of a bypass operation. The third part of the duodenum is exposed by an incision through the parietal peritoneum of the posterior abdominal wall, after the transverse colon and its mesocolon have been turned upward. The posterior parietal peritoneum is reflected and the retroperitoneal areolar tissue in front of the anterior aspect of the duodenum is dissected away. The prestenotic portion of the duodenum to the right of the superior mesenteric vessels is then connected in a site-to-site anastomosis with the proximal jejunum, thus bypassing the obstructed area.

26 Liver Abscess with Rupture into Lung

A 37-year-old geologist, who has spent the last twelve years in Central and South America working for an oil company, is referred to the hospital by his physician with the diagnosis of chronic intestinal amebiasis. His symptoms gradually started several years ago and consisted of intermittent attacks of diarrhea with abdominal discomfort and five to ten stools daily. In spite of this, he had good appetite and continued to work. Slowly, his symptoms worsened. He lost a great deal of weight and became disabled. A diagnosis of amebic dysentery was made and he was sent back to the States. He now complains of loss of appetite, frequent abdominal cramps, and numerous bloody stools. His pain is particularly noticeable in the right upper abdomen and lower chest with extension into the right shoulder and neck. The pain in the lower part of the right chest is quite severe and is aggravated by deep inspiration. Recently he also developed a cough leading to expectoration of large quantities of reddish-brown, bloody sputum.

EXAMINATION

On examination we find a patient in poor nutritional state who appears listless and quite ill. He seems dehydrated and his temperature reaches a peak of 101°. On palpation, the whole abdomen is quite sore, but there is particular tenderness in the right hypochondriac region. The liver is enlarged and palpable three inches below the right costal margin.

Pressure by the examining fingertips over the anterior lower right intercostal spaces indicates an area which is particularly tender and corresponds to the convexity of the right lobe of the liver. On percussion and auscultation of the lungs there are signs of immobility of the right diaphragm and of marked lung involvement with numerous rales and dullness on percussion. The white count is quite elevated. The dark-reddish sputum contains the organism responsible for amebic dysentery, *Entamoeba histolytica.* Sigmoidoscopic examination reveals amebic ulcers with hyperemia and edema of the mucosa. Blood-stained muscus is recovered in which typical motile amebae can be demonstrated. Fluoroscopy and roentgenography show elevation and immobilization of the right diaphragm and consolidation of the lower medial portions of the right lung field. There is an abscess cavity demonstrable, which on profile view can be placed in the right middle lobe.

Under local anesthesia and careful aseptic conditions, puncture of the liver at its most painful area is done and pus aspirated by syringe. The material obtained consists of a paste-like, brownish substance which on microscopic examination is identified as necrotic liver tissue, red cells and some pus cells, and pathogenic amebae.

DIAGNOSIS

Amebic intestinal dysentery with an hepatic abscess, which has ruptured into the middle lobe of the right lung.

THERAPY AND FURTHER COURSE

The puncture of the liver and aspiration of its abscess relieves the pain and greatly improves the patient's clinical condition. He is put on narcotics, sedatives, and bedrest and receives frequent small feedings of a high protein diet and adequate fluids. The patient is immediately started on specific chemotherapy with emetine and chloroquine. A broad spectrum antibiotic is also given to prevent bacterial superinfection. Under this treatment the patient improves rapidly, the enlargement

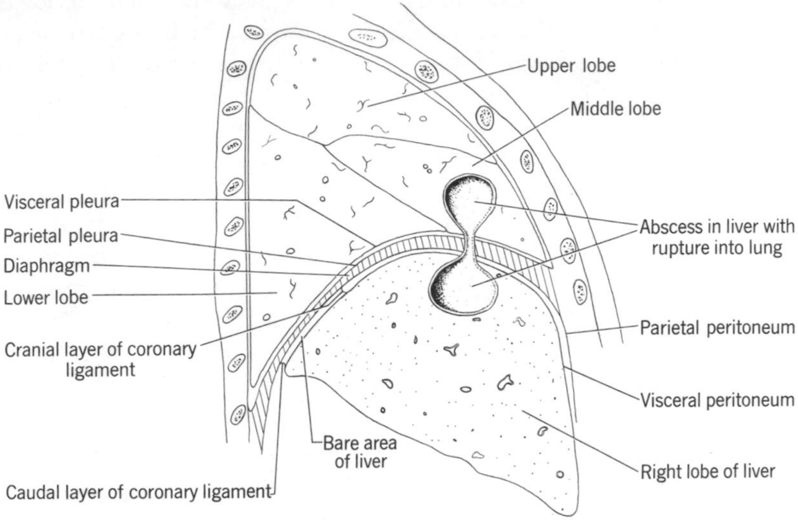

Figure 1—Profile view of right lung and liver in a parasagittal plane shows abcess cavity in the convexity of right lobe of liver that has ruptured into the middle lobe of the right lung, causing a daughter-abscess.

of the liver gradually subsides, and his appetite increases. The pain disappears and his cough ceases. On the roentgenogram only pleural scarring can now be demonstrated. After two weeks, three stool examinations for amebae are negative and the patient is discharged for home care. A reexamination six months later shows the patient well and without gastrointestinal symptoms. He has gained twenty-five pounds and has returned to his former position.

DISCUSSION

Mode of spread of amebic infection to the liver

This patient has a chronic ulcerative disease of the large intestine, which is caused by an ameba, the *Entamoeba histolytica*. He acquired this disease in the tropics where it is more frequent than in the United States. How does this lesion of the colon spread to the liver? It is known that amebae enter the capillaries and venules of the submucosa and muscularis of the colon, where they can be demonstrated. What is the venous drainage of the colon? The superior mesenteric vein drains, in addition to parts of the stomach, pancreas, and small intestine, the cecum, appendix, ascending colon, and transverse colon. The cecum, appendix, and ascending colon are favorite sites of amebic dysentery. The inferior mesenteric vein drains the rest of the large intestine. Here sigmoid colon and rectum are frequently involved in the disease. Both veins, together with the splenic, form the portal vein, which then branches like an artery to terminate in the sinusoids of the liver. By this pathway, the amebae are brought to the liver, where they may cause hepatic necrosis and abscess cavities. Typically, these amebic abscesses are single and occur most frequently in the right lobe near the dome of the liver. This was also the location of the hepatic abscess in our patient.

Mode of spread of hepatic abscess to the lung

How do you explain the involvement of the lung in our case and the absence of peritoneal infection? The amebic infection of the lung is the result of direct extension of the liver abscess into the lung. How many layers of serous membranes have to be traversed by rupture of the hepatic abscess into the lung? Two layers of peritoneum and two layers of pleura are eroded by the pus from the hepatic abscess. Identify these layers. They are the visceral peritoneal layer covering the dome of the liver, the parietal layer of the peritoneum lining the undersurface of the adjacent diaphragm, the diaphragmatic part of the parietal pleura, and the visceral pleura covering the base of the right lung (Fig. 1).

How can you explain the non-involvement of the free peritoneal and pleural cavities in our case? As so often happens when the hepatic abscess enlarges, it approaches the diaphragm and causes formation of adhesions between the visceral peritoneum covering the abscess and the parietal peritoneal lining of the diaphragm. Slow development of the penetration of the diaphragm also allows pleural adhesions to form between its parietal and visceral layers. Thus, the general peritoneal and pleural cavities are sealed off at the site of the hepatic abscess, which then breaks through into the lung.

Site of lung abscess

What is the site of the secondary abscess in the lung? It is located in the right middle lobe. Later, breakthrough into a bronchus allows part of the pus from the lung abscess to be expectorated. How do you explain the fact that the middle lobe and not the lower lobe is involved in this rupture into the base of the lung? The student is inclined to think of the lobes of the lung as vertically stacked tiers, the superior being cranial to the middle lobe and the latter cranial to the inferior lobe, with only the inferior lobe forming the base of the lung. This is erroneous. While it is probably too late to change the firmly entrenched and historically reinforced terminology of the lobes, it would be wise to think of them as anterosuperior, anteromiddle, and posteroinferior lobes. Thus, the middle lobe forms the anterior part of the base of the lung and both inferior and middle lobes are in contact with the diaphragm with only pleura intervening (Fig. 1).

What segments form the base of the lung?

Give the total number of pulmonary segments that form the base of the right lung. Six segments participate in the base: the lateral and medial segments of the middle lobe, and the medial, anterior, lateral, and posterior basal segments of the inferior lobe (Fig. 2).

Which segments of the left lung are in contact with the diaphragm with only pleura intervening? It is often not realized that, in addition to the basal segments of the inferior lobe, the inferior segment of the lingular portion of the left superior lobe also reaches the diaphragm, although only

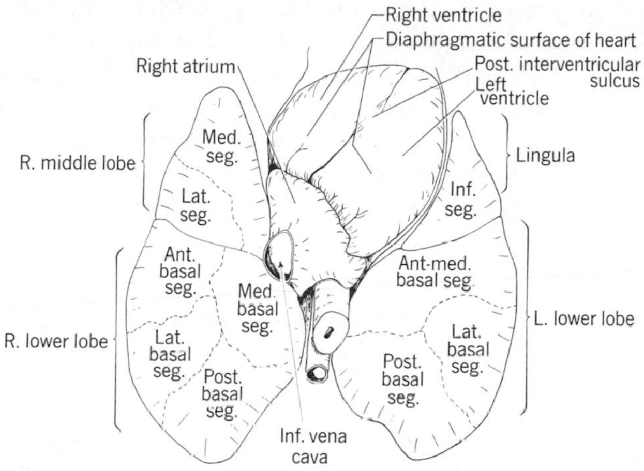

Figure 2—Basal view of the diaphragmatic surfaces of both lungs and heart, showing the individual segments of middle and lower lobes on the right, and upper and lower lobes on the left that are in contact with the diaphragm, only pleura intervening. Notice that both segments of the middle lobe and four basal segments of the right lower lobe have a diaphragmatic aspect. Observe particularly that the left upper lobe with its inferior segment of the lingula also borders on the diaphragm. In addition, three or four basal segments of the left lower lobe have a diaphragmatic surface.

in a small area. Theoretically it is conceivable, but not very probable, that abscesses of the left lobe of the liver may extend directly into this segment of the left superior lobe (Fig. 2).

Homologies of right and left lungs

The oblique fissure divides the left lung in two lobes which, from their location and spatial relationship, might have been more appropriately identified as anterosuperior and posteroinferior lobes, rather than as superior and inferior lobes. Of what portion of the left lung is the right middle lobe a homologue? By bronchial similarities, location, and by the occasional presence of a horizontal fissure on the left, the right middle lobe and the lower part of the left superior lobe are regarded as homologous. This portion of the left lung is called the lingula (little tongue) and its bronchus is the inferior (lingular) division of the superior lobe bronchus. What is the homologue of the left superior lobe on the right? The right superior and middle lobes together correspond to the left superior lobe.

Perforation of amebic abscess into serous cavities, adjacent organs and structures

If the destructive process in the liver is more acute, the abscess may rupture without adhesions having been formed to wall it off. In this case, the abscess may break through into the pleural or peritoneal cavities causing dangerous infection in these spaces. On occasion, an amebic abscess of the liver ruptures into the pericardium, causing a suppurative (pus-producing) and generally fatal pericarditis. In which lobe of the liver is such an abscess most likely located? It is the left lobe of the liver which underlies the pericardial sac and from which abscesses may perforate into this cavity.

Can you visualize a liver abscess rupturing into the abdominal cavity and causing a subphrenic abscess without involvement of the peritoneal cavity? Perforation through the bare area of the liver results in such an extraperitoneal subphrenic abscess. This complication is not infrequent. The literature lists rarer perforations of a liver abscess into the following organs and structures: stomach, duodenum, small and large intestines, spleen, inferior vena cava, right renal pelvis, and through the skin to the outside. All these structures are in close relation to the liver and may be anchored to the site of the abscess by previously formed adhesions.

Pain pathways involved in this case

Additional interest centers on the anatomical pathways responsible for the pain-pattern in our patient. In the case history we notice that he complains of pain in the right hypochondriac region and in the right lower chest. The pain increases in deep inspiration and radiates into the right neck and shoulder. Tenderness on digital pressure is quite marked in the thoracic and abdominal walls overlying the liver.

In defining the anatomical pain pathways involved, we have to realize that visceral pleura and visceral peritoneum are insensitive to pain. There are then essentially three channels along which painful sensations travel in our case. Visceral pain is due to stretching of the capsule of the liver. This pain is mediated through afferent fibers of the sympathetic system that accompany the efferent fibers. The afferent fibers course by way of the hepatic plexus in the free margin of the lesser omentum and pass without synapse through the celiac ganglia, greater and lesser splanchnic nerves, thoracic sympathetic chain ganglia, white rami communicantes, spinal nerves and then by way of the posterior roots to spinal ganglia T6 to T10. Here their cell bodies are located and the centrally directed fibers of the ganglia reach the spinal cord.

On the other hand, the pain in the thoracic and abdominal walls, including their serous linings, is somatic sensory in character and is mediated by the sensory component of the intercostal nerves which supply the body wall of this region. It is this pain which is increased by digital pressure. In contrast to their visceral portions, the parietal layers of peritoneum and pleura are quite sensitive to pain and irritated in our case by the underlying infection of liver and lung.

A third component of our patient's pain-pattern is mediated through the phrenic nerve which, in addition to its well-known motor function, supplies the diaphragmatic portion of the parietal peritoneum, the diaphragm, and the central part of the diaphragmatic pleura (also the pericardium and mediastinal pleura). This type of pain is frequently referred to neck and shoulder. One explanation often given for the phenomenon of pain referral is that pain arising in the interior of the body, and particularly in the viscera, is interpreted as coming from that area of the body surface which sends sensory impulses to the same segments of the cord that receive visceral sensation. The phrenic nerve arises from cervical segments three, four, and five which also supply the periphery of neck and shoulder with sensory fibers by way of the great auricular and supraclavicular nerves. These nerves are the mediators of referred pain in our patient.

27 Appendicitis

A 22-year-old male university student and collegiate athlete, who has been in excellent health, was suddenly seized in the middle of the night by a severe attack of "indigestion" accompanied by cramp like pains above and around the umbilicus. He tried to move his bowels but did not succeed. Next morning he felt hot and uncomfortable and decided to stay in bed. He had no appetite and some nausea and did not eat anything. By evening the pain had then moved to the right lower abdominal region. He consulted a physician, who transferred him to a hospital.

EXAMINATION

On examination the patient lies on his back with his right thigh flexed. He has a slightly increased temperature of 99.6°; his pulse rate is somewhat elevated. The patient now localizes his pain in the right lower abdominal region. On palpation of the abdomen there is marked localized tenderness and some rigidity in the right iliac fossa. On pressure with the fingertip the area of greatest tenderness is located near McBurney's point (Fig. 1). On rectal examination there is a definite difference in sensitivity in palpating the right and left sides of the rectovesical pouch: the right side is distinctly more tender.

DIAGNOSIS

The typical history of acute onset with loss of appetite, nausea, and constipation, and the change in the site of pain from the epigastric and umbilical to the right iliac region, make the diagnosis of acute appendicitis most likely. This is confirmed by the localized tenderness elicited on the abdomen and by rectal examination.

THERAPY

In view of the diagnosis of acute appendicitis, and in order to forestall complications such as perforation and peritonitis, immediate operation is advised and performed.

A right lower muscle-splitting incision through the abdominal wall is chosen to obtain access to the appendix. In this incision the external and internal abdominal oblique muscles and the transverse abdominis muscles and their aponeuroses are split in the direction of their fibers. Next the transversalis fascia, the extraperitoneal fat, and the parietal peritoneum are incised, and the appendix is visualized. In our case the appendix is found to be greatly inflamed and distended, and its visceral peritoneal covering is quite red. The appendix crosses the psoas major muscle and reaches into the true pelvis with its tip hanging over the pelvic brim. It is raised and delivered into the wound.

The mesenteriolum of the appendix is clamped and divided and the appendicular vessels and their branches are ligated. Next the base (root) of the appendix is clamped, crushed, and ligated, and the appendix amputated distal to the ligature. The stump of the appendix is cauterized, inverted and buried by sutures within the wall of the cecum. The peritoneum and the other components of the abdominal wall are closed in layers.

FURTHER COURSE

Under administration of intravenous fluids and antibiotics the patient progresses satisfactorily and is discharged from the hospital six days after operation.

DISCUSSION

Appendicitis is generally brought about by occlusion of the lumen of the appendix vermiformis by a fecal stone or by some food particle, with subsequent distension of the blind sac distal to the obstruction. Infection and inflammation develop in the distended portion. This may lead to tissue death, perforation, and abscess formation. What features in the anatomy of the appendix predispose the organ to inflammation and rupture? The appendix has often been called the "tonsil of the abdomen," which refers to the accumulation of lymphatic tissue within its wall and the proneness to infection. The absence of a well-developed muscular coat facilitates perforation and spread of infection to the serosa.

Anatomy of pain transmission in appendicitis

How can the changing pattern of pain, shifting from the region of the umbilicus to the right iliac area, be explained? The initial pain in the epigastric and umbilical regions originates in visceral sensory fibers in the wall of the inflamed appendix. What is the course of these sensory fibers? Where are their cell bodies located?

The sensory impulses from the appendix travel in visceral sensory fibers, which are closely intermingled with sympathetic efferent fibers, through collateral ganglia, splanchnic nerves, and chain ganglia, and via white rami communicantes to spinal nerves and their posterior roots and ganglia. Here their cell bodies are located. Central fibers from these ganglion cells continue into the spinal cord. For physiologic reasons the pain arising in the appendiceal wall is referred to areas of the body surface which send sensory impulses to the same segments of the cord that receive pain impulses from the appendix, that is, supposedly ninth thoracic to first lumbar. What segment of the spinal cord is mainly responsible for the innervation of the skin area around the umbilicus? The tenth thoracic cord segment supplies the area around the umbilicus with overlap from the ninth and eleventh segments.

The later pain in the right iliac region seems to be caused

by stimulation of somatic sensory fibers supplying the parietal peritoneum of the abdominal wall. What spinal nerves carrying somatic sensory fibers from the abdominal wall are involved in transmission of this type of pain? The lowest intercostal, the subcostal, and the first lumbar nerves carry somatic sensory (pain) fibers from this area. Tenderness of palpation and the protective muscle contraction, which expresses itself as rigidity of the right lateral abdominal wall, are likewise the result of irritation of the parietal peritoneum.

McBurney's point

What is the location of McBurney's point? It is classically defined as a point two inches from the right anterior superior iliac spine upon a line joining this spine with the umbilicus (Fig. 1). As originally conceived by McBurney, this point is supposed to correspond to the site of origin of the appendix. But variability in the position of the umbilicus, in the degree of descent of the cecum, and in the location of the origin of the appendix makes this point a somewhat questionable landmark.

Positive psoas test and rectal findings

How do you explain the preference of the patient for flexion of the thigh? What muscle is a posterior relation of the appendix and also a flexor of the thigh? In our case the appendix crosses the psoas major muscle and the patient prefers flexion of the thigh to relieve tension of the inflamed area (Fig. 1). The opposite movement, hyperextension of the thigh, puts the psoas muscle and its inflamed fascia on the stretch and is painful and resisted by the patient (psoas test in appendicitis).

What is the explanation for the difference in sensitivity on rectal examination in palpating the right and left sides of the rectovesical pouch? Define the latter pouch. It is the outpouching of the caudalmost extent of the peritoneal cavity between bladder and rectum in the male. The increased tenderness on

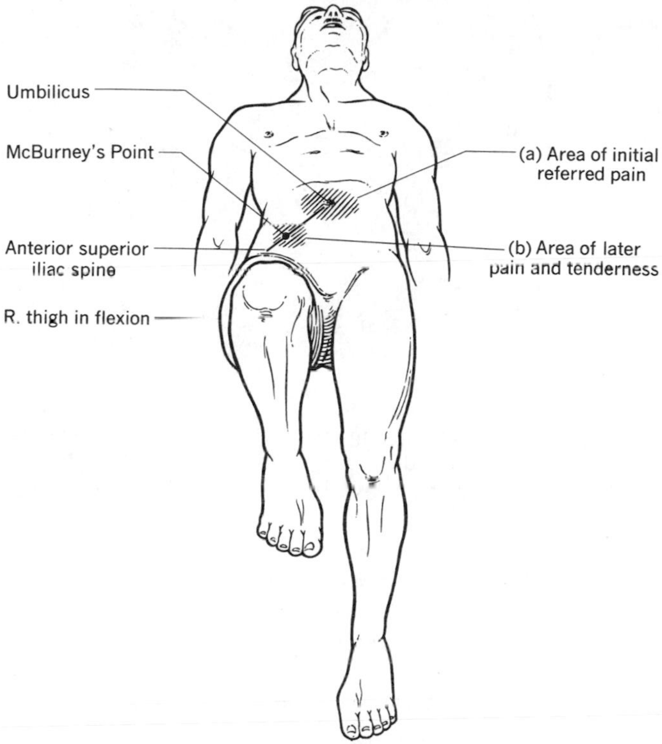

Figure 1—The two areas of pain: (a) initial referred pain in the umbilical and para-umbilical region; (b) later pain in the right iliac region due to irritation of the parietal peritoneum. McBurney's point is at the site of greatest tenderness. Thigh is flexed to relieve tension.

the right side of this pouch indicates irritation or inflammation of the parietal peritoneum in this area.

Anatomy of the right lower abdominal muscle-splitting incision

The approach to the appendix in this case was a right lower abdominal muscle-splitting incision through the abdominal wall. What is the direction of the fibers of the three lateral abdominal muscles in this area? The fibers of the external

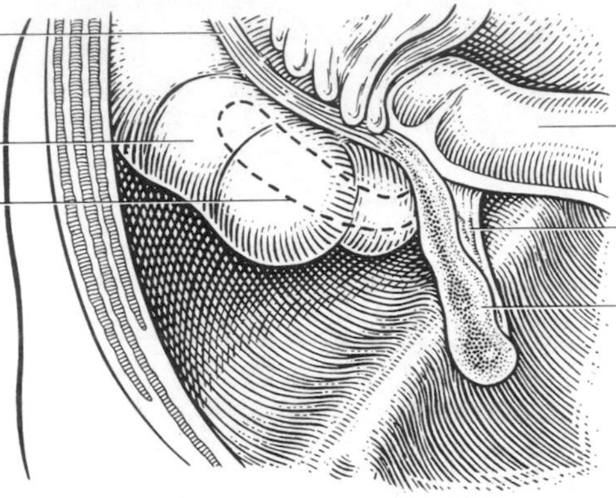

Figure 2—Appendix vermiformis is inflamed and distended in its distal portion with its tip hanging over the pelvic brim. Notice how the ventral taenia acts as a guide to the origin of the appendix. Notice also how a retrocecal appendix might be difficult to approach surgically.

abdominal oblique muscle run from lateral above to medial below ("as if you put your hand in your front pocket"). What is the direction of the fibers of the internal abdominal oblique and transversus abdominis muscles in the right iliac region? The fibers of both muscles generally run transversely in this area. What is the direction of the fibers of the internal oblique muscle somewhat more cranially? They run at right angles to the external oblique fibers ("as if you put your hand in your back pocket"). Care must be taken not to injure what important nerves that lie deep to the internal oblique muscle in the operative field? The iliohypogastric and ilioinguinal nerves may be damaged by this incision.

Location of appendix. Its blood supply

What arrangement in the longitudinal musculature of the cecum assists in locating the origin of the appendix (Fig. 2)? The ventral taenia forms the best guide to this point.

In our case the position of the appendix facilitated its removal. What common location of the appendix would be apt to cause technical difficulties at the time of surgery? Retrocecal position of the appendix could make the operation more difficult.

What blood vessels are ligated in the mesenteriolum of the appendix? The blood vessels that are ligated are the appendicular artery and vein and their branches and tributaries. Of what artery is the appendicular artery usually a branch, and how does it run in relation to the last part of the ileum? The appendicular artery generally is a branch of the ileocolic artery from the superior mesenteric artery and passes posterior to the terminal portion of the ileum to enter the mesenteriolum of the appendix.

Identify the named veins through which an ascending infection in the appendicular vein would have to pass to reach the liver and cause liver abscesses. The infection would travel by way of the appendicular, ileocolic, superior mesenteric, and portal veins to the liver.

28 Hydronephrosis due to Aberrant Renal Vessel

A five-year-old girl is brought to a physician's office with a history of periodic febrile attacks and complaints of intermittent sharp pain in the left loin. The mother states that the attacks occurred every few months and lasted one or two days. They were accompanied by nausea and vomiting. She also complains that the child eats poorly and that she has not gained any weight during the last eight months. The patient is admitted to the Children's Hospital for further study.

EXAMINATION

The physical examination shows a rather poorly nourished, but normally developed child with a slightly enlarged and tender left kidney. Urine examination reveals numerous pus cells. Her temperature is 99.6° and her white count is elevated.

The patient is roentgenographed, and an X-ray opaque dye that is excreted by the kidney is injected intravenously. The roentgenogram of the kidneys with the opacified pelves and calices shows a moderate enlargement of the left pelvis and calices. The right kidney appears normal. Under local anesthesia the girl is cystoscoped and catheters inserted into both ureters. The urine flowing from the right ureter is clear, while the urine on the left is cloudy and contains pus. The catheter on the left is then inserted into the pelvis of the kidney and 10 cc. of an X-ray opaque medium are injected in order to visualize the pelvis and calices. After withdrawal of the

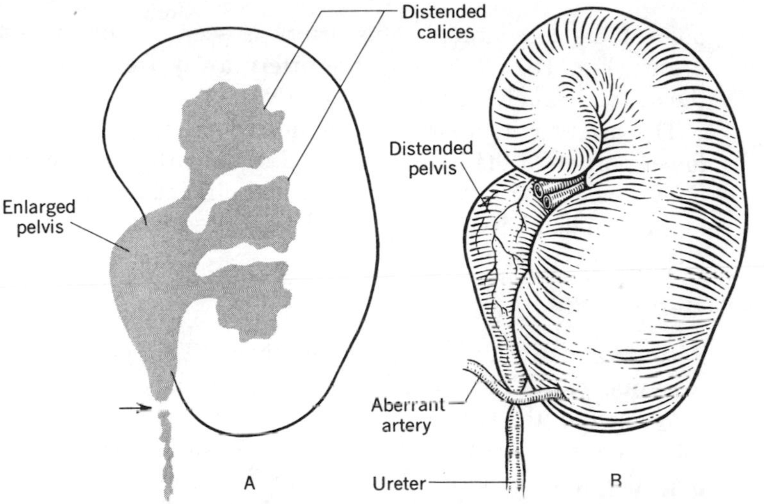

Figure 1A.—Roentgenogram of the left kidney shows dilated renal pelvis and calices and an indentation of the ureter at the ureteropelvic junction (see arrow). 1B.—Diagram shows the enlarged kidney with an accessory (aberrant) artery going to the lower pole and indenting and compressing the left ureter.

catheter into the lower portion of the left ureter, further injection of contrast medium demonstrates the ureter. Roentgen films of the left urinary tract taken at various stages of the procedure show a dilated renal pelvis and calices and a distinct indentation and narrowing at the ureteropelvic junction (Fig. 1A).

DIAGNOSIS

Moderate hydronephrosis (dilatation of pelvis and calices) of the left kidney with obstruction at the ureteropelvic junction, possibly due to an aberrant blood vessel.

THERAPY

The patient is operated. At operation the left kidney appears enlarged and the pelvis bulging. An accessory artery is seen to pass from the aorta in front of the left ureter to the lower pole of the left kidney. This artery is seen to compress the ureter (Fig. 1B). On easing the artery away from the ureter the distended pelvis empties promptly.

The artery is temporarily compressed, and the area of the lower portion of the kidney supplied by the artery is inspected. Only a slight discoloration is noticed, which lasts only a few minutes. The aberrant artery is then ligated and divided.

FURTHER COURSE

Postoperatively, antibiotics were given. The convalescence was uneventful. Periodic urinalysis showed continuous improvement of the kidney infection. Serial roentgen studies with intravenous application of dye at six-month intervals revealed that the kidney and calices gradually returned to a more normal size and capacity. Two years later the mother reported that the child was well and without complaints.

DISCUSSION

Aberrant renal vessels to the inferior pole of the kidney occur in 4 to 6 per cent of all kidneys and may be a cause of obstruction of the upper urinary tract. How do you explain, from an embryological point of view, the appearance of supernumerary renal arteries at levels different from the main renal artery? Where during fetal development are the kidneys located and how do they reach their definitive location in the lumbar region? The kidneys develop originally in the pelvis and migrate from there cranially by gradual retroperitoneal ascent. While they are located in the pelvis, they are supplied by blood vessels in the neighborhood originating from the common, external, or internal iliac arteries, the inferior mesenteric artery, or aorta. Most of the these regional vessels disappear as the kidneys ascend, but some may persist as supernumerary or aberrant arteries supplying portions of the kidney, particularly the lower pole.

What is the clinical importance of this anomaly? In crossing the ureter, more commonly anteriorly than posteriorly, these aberrant vessels may cause an intermittent or continuous obstruction to urinary drainage from the pelvis. How do you explain the progressive enlargement of the renal pelvis and calices (hydronephrosis) and the eventual destruction of the renal cortex in these cases? Pressure of the backed-up urine may gradually distend and enlarge the pelvis and calices of the kidney and destroy the cortex. An important factor in this progressive destruction of the kidney is the interference with the intrarenal blood supply by increased intrarenal pressure. What is the cause for the frequently superimposed infection of the kidney? The insufficiently nourished and diseased kidney with its stagnating urine may readily become the site of blood-borne infection originating in the upper respiratory tract or elsewhere.

What is the clinical significance of the accessory arteries to the *upper pole* of the kidney and from what arteries are they derived? They may be inadvertently torn in renal surgery leading to severe or sometimes fatal hemorrhage. They are most commonly derived from phrenic or suprarenal arteries. What in the X-ray findings in our case pointed to the diagnosis of an aberrant vessel as the cause of hydronephrosis? The indentation and narrowing of the ureter just caudal to the enlarged pelvis was certainly significant.

To what extent would ligation of an accessory polar renal artery interfere with the blood supply to the kidney? This is a serious problem in the design of surgery for the condition under discussion since severance of a major artery to the kidney would entail loss of function of that portion of the kidney supplied by the artery and may result in renal necrosis and infection. If the amount of renal parenchyma involved is more than one-fourth of the organ, the artery should be left intact and circumvented by plastic surgery that establishes a junction of the ureter and pelvis unencumbered by the aberrant artery. Temporary compression of the artery at the time of surgery and observation of resulting color changes in the area of the kidney supplied by the artery will furnish a clue to the importance of the artery.

Other causes of ureteral obstruction

Is it possible that the crossing of the ureter by the aberrant artery is not the primary cause of the obstruction, but coincides with some internal stenosis of the ureter at the same site and acts only as a contributing factor on an already enlarged pelvis that is sagging caudally over the accessory vessel? This hypothesis has been put forth in the literature by a number of authors who ascribe the primary intraureteral stenosis to congenital mucosal valves or inherent narrowing of the ureter. Such malformations certainly do occur as a cause of hydronephrosis and not all supernumerary lower polar vessels cause obstruction of the ureter. Consequently, the ureter must be opened at the time of surgery if there is a suspicion of an internal stenosis. In that case, plastic surgery of the ureter is indicated.

29 Prolapse of the Uterus

A farmer's wife, 42 years old, comes to the out-patient department with the following complaints. She has a bearing down sensation in her womb, "something seems to come down." This discomfort increases when she strains or lifts heavy loads. She often has backaches, particularly if she is on her feet all day. She also complains of urinary symptoms, such as frequency of and burning on urination. She fatigues easily. The patient has had four children and two miscarriages. Her menstrual flow is increased and her periods are somewhat irregular.

EXAMINATION

On general examination the patient appears nervous and anxious. She is underweight and rather frail. Otherwise the general examination does not show any abnormalities.

Gynecological examination reveals a moderate downward bulging of the anterior vaginal wall which increases on straining. On examination in the erect position the cervix of the uterus is found in the vagina close to the vestibule. It recedes somewhat when the patient is supine, yet does not assume its normal position. The cervix is elongated (Fig. 1).

DIAGNOSIS

Prolapse (descensus or downward displacement) of the uterus into the vagina and cystocele (bulging of the bladder into the anterior vaginal wall).

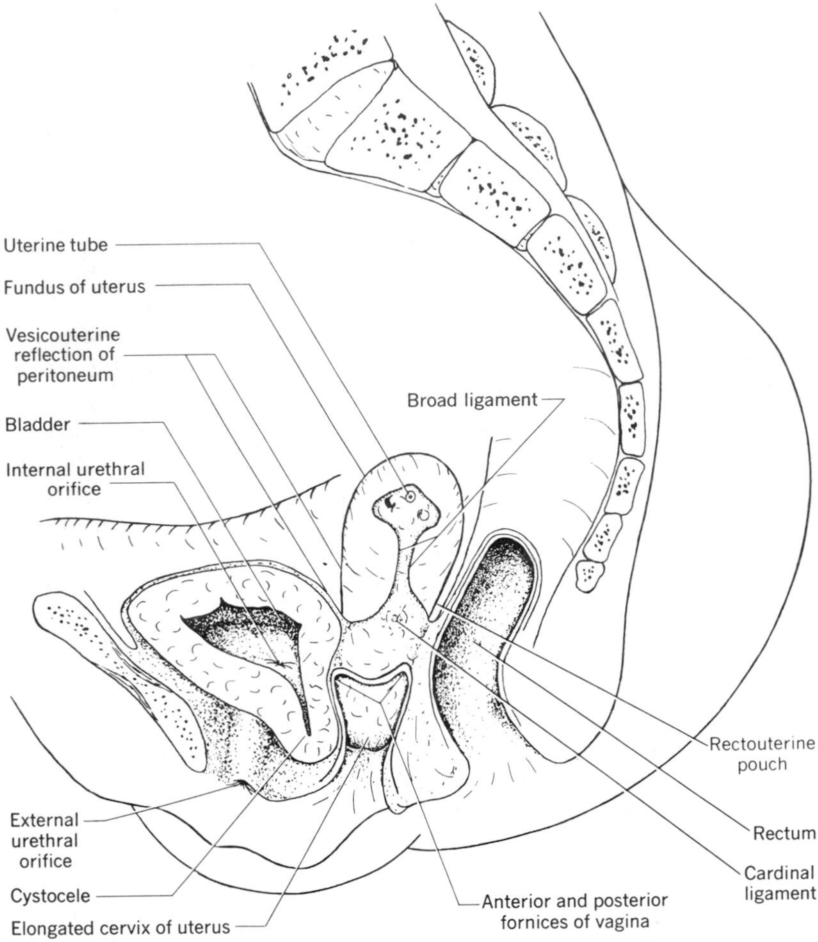

Figure 1 shows prolapse of the uterus and cystocele. Notice the retroverted position of the partially descended uterus and the elongation of the cervix. Observe the bulging of the bladder into the anterior vaginal wall.

THERAPY AND FURTHER COURSE

Since the patient is otherwise in good health and relatively young, though frail, reconstructive surgery is recommended and agreed upon. Under general anesthesia the patient is placed in the lithotomy position (that is, the legs are flexed on the thighs, and the thighs flexed on the abdomen and abducted). Traction on the cervix near its os brings the cervix and the everted mucosa of the anterior vaginal wall into the operative field. The anterior vaginal wall is split by a longitudinal inverted T-shaped midline incision, and the fascial plane between bladder and cervix/vagina is reached. By alternating blunt and sharp dissection the bladder is separated from the cervix up to the vesicouterine reflection of the peritoneum. The cardinal ligaments are exposed and cut at their attachment to the cervix. The cervical branches of the uterine artery are ligated and divided.

A circular incision is made around the lower portion of the cervix and this portion is amputated. The cut ends of the cardinal ligaments are shortened and sutured in front of the stump of the cervix. The vesicovaginal fascia and the perivesical connective tissue is pleated and firmly sutured over the new attachment of the cardinal ligaments to support the bladder-neck and the floor of the bladder. The stump of the cervix is covered with mucosal flaps and the cut surface in the vaginal mucosa is closed by sutures after portions of redundant mucosa have been excised.

Postoperatively the patient is catheterized every four to six hours and receives antibiotics. Warm, moist applications and dry heat are applied to the perineum. Catheterization is discontinued after three days, and the patient is discharged from the hospital one week after operation.

Reexamination after three and six months does not show any recurrence of the prolapse.

DISCUSSION

Uterine prolapse often combined with a cystocele, as we find it in our patient, is one of the most frequently encountered gynecological disorders. What is the cause of the uterine prolapse and the cystocele? With advancing age there is increased relaxation and loss of tonus of the muscular and fascial structures that constitute the support of the pelvic viscera. This fact is mainly responsible for the disorder. Do multiple childbirths contribute to the occurrence of uterine prolapse? Lacerations and overstretching of the supporting tissues during childbirth greatly enhance the chances for prolapse.

How do you explain the discomfort of the patient, consisting of a feeling of heaviness in the lower abdomen and backache? These seem to be due to venous congestion and traction on the ligaments of the uterus by the pull of the prolapsed organ.

How do you explain the urinary symptoms such as frequency and burning in cystocele? Due to the dislodgment of the bladder residual urine remains in the bladder after urination resulting in periodic infection of the stagnating urine and cystitis. Frequency and burning are typical signs of this disorder.

Flexion and version of the uterus

What is the normal position of the uterus? What angles do the terms "version" and "flexion" pertaining to the uterus indicate? The uterus is a very mobile organ, subject to constant changes in its position depending on the state of filling of the organs in its neighborhood, that is, mainly bladder and rectum. With these organs empty or nearly empty, the most common position of the uterus is that of anteversion denoting an anteriorly open angle of somewhat more than 90° between the long axes of the uterus and vagina. In addition the uterus is generally also anteflexed, which denotes an anteriorly open angle between uterine body and cervix. When the bladder fills, the uterus is readily elevated or even retroverted by the upper surface of the bladder, while filling of the rectum may increase its anteversion and anteflexion (Fig. 2). In what direction does the ostium of the uterus face if the uterus is in its typical anteverted position? It opens posteriorly into the

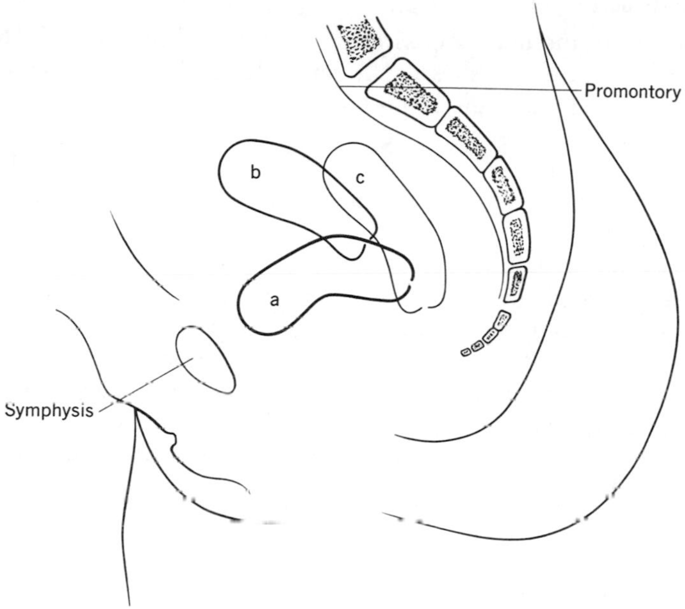

Figure 2 demonstrates the variable position of the uterus in the pelvis depending on the state of filling of the rectum and bladder. Position of the uterus (a) with bladder and rectum empty; (b) with bladder and rectum filled; (c) with full bladder and empty rectum (after Merkel).

vagina. On the other hand, the uterine opening faces anteriorly if the uterus is retroverted.

In contrast to former teaching, retroversion and retroflexion by themselves are of questionable clinical significance. If uterine supports are weakened, a retroverted and retroflexed position of the uterus tends to promote descent of the uterus since it then lies in the extension of the longitudinal axis of the vagina (Fig. 1). Intra-abdominal pressure further accentuates the downward displacement of the cervix. Congestion and swelling gradually result in elongation of the cervix as in our patient.

Uterine support

What are the main supporting structures of the uterus? Here the literature furnishes conflicting information, disagreeing in the evaluation of the importance of various structures.

The principal support of the uterus is the pelvic diaphragm which with its fascial coverings forms the fibromuscular floor of the pelvis. What is the main muscular constituent of the pelvic diaphragm? The levator ani closes the pelvis caudally. It is variable in thickness and is often partly replaced by connective tissue after having been lacerated and stretched during childbirth. Its two halves are separated in front by a narrow gap. Give the name of the gap and state what partially closes it. The genital hiatus in front of the anal canal transmits the vagina and urethra and is partially obliterated by the urogenital diaphragm. The importance of the levator ani for the support of the uterus is exemplified by cases where, due to congenital paralysis of the levator ani in malformations of the spinal cord, there is already a prolapse of the uterus in the early years of childhood. The support of the uterus by the levator ani and the urogenital diaphragm is mainly indirect, however, in that the uterus rests on organs which on their part are sustained in their position by the intact pelvic and urogenital diaphragms. These organs are the bladder, on which the normally anteverted and anteflexed uterus rests, and the ampulla of the rectum, which supports the cervix uteri and the vagina caudally and posteriorly.

Particularly controversial is the role of the cardinal (lateral cervical) ligaments. Define these ligaments. They are condensations of parametrial connective tissue in the base of the broad ligaments, around and caudal to the uterine vessels. The cardinal ligaments extend from the lateral pelvic wall to the cervix and upper part of the vagina. Questionable and variable is the amount of smooth musculature, if any, that they contain.

Finally the fibrous connective tissue between the vagina and bladder and vagina and urethra should be mentioned as a supporting factor. The former is loosely areolar, the latter denser. Clinicians have given them the names of vesicovaginal and urethrovaginal septa or fasciae. They are a part of the pelvic visceral fascia and fuse with the outer layers of the organs previously mentioned.

Applied anatomy of prolapse surgery

What is the rationale of the operation for uterine prolapse and cystocele utilized in this case? During surgery the dislodged viscera are replaced back to their original position and the potential space between bladder and vagina, through which the bladder prolapsed, is obliterated by sutures and a firm support given to the bladder. The overstretched and redundant vaginal wall is partially resected and repaired. The elongated portion of the cervix is resected, thus decreasing the pull and weight on the body of the uterus. The shortening and attachment of the medial ends of the cardinal ligaments in front of the cervical stump assure normal posterior direction of the cervix and uterine os and therefore an anteflexed and anteverted position of the uterine body, making the latter rest on the bladder.

When there is a weakness of the posterior vaginal wall with bulging of the rectum through this wall (rectocele), the stretched portions of the levator ani are likewise repaired and brought together, thus strengthening the pelvic diaphragm. Occasionally the rectouterine ligaments lying within the rectouterine peritoneal folds are also shortened to assure a posterior pull on the cervix and an anterior rotation of the body of the uterus.

What important structures are endangered when the cardinal ligaments are shortened? What is the position of these structures in relation to the uterus and the uterine artery? The ureters are usually somewhat displaced in uterine prolapse. Great care should be exercised during the division of the cardinal ligaments to prevent damage to the ureters. In their anteriorly and medialward directed course toward the bladder, they pass by the sides of the cervix and lateral fornices of the vagina at a distance of only 1 to 2 cm. Here they are closely related to the cardinal ligaments at the base of the broad ligaments. The uterine artery crosses cranially and in front of the ureter ("water runs under the bridge"), giving a small branch to it. The ureter may be mistaken for the uterine artery and erroneously ligated in surgical removal of the uterus.

30 Vasectomy

A 32-year-old geologist had a vasectomy (excision of a segment of the vas or ductus deferens) five years earlier for the purpose of sterilization, his wife having undergone three Caesarian sections. In the meantime he has remarried and his second wife desires children of her own. He consults a urologist to find out whether reunion of the deferent ducts could be done. The urologist recommends the operation but does not promise success.

THERAPY

Under general anesthesia an incision into the scrotum is made at the site of the former operation. Puncture of the epididymis verifies the presence of active spermatozoa. Both ends of the ligated ductus deferens are freed for 2 cm and brought to the surface. They are freshened to the point where patency can be observed. Then an end-to-end anastomosis is established with all layers of the duct being properly approximated. The duct of the opposite side is repaired in the same manner. The incisions are closed and a suspensory (support) is prescribed to immobilize the scrotal contents.

Laboratory studies on two occasions within the next months prove the presence of live spermatozoa in the semen. Six months later the patient reports that his wife has become pregnant.

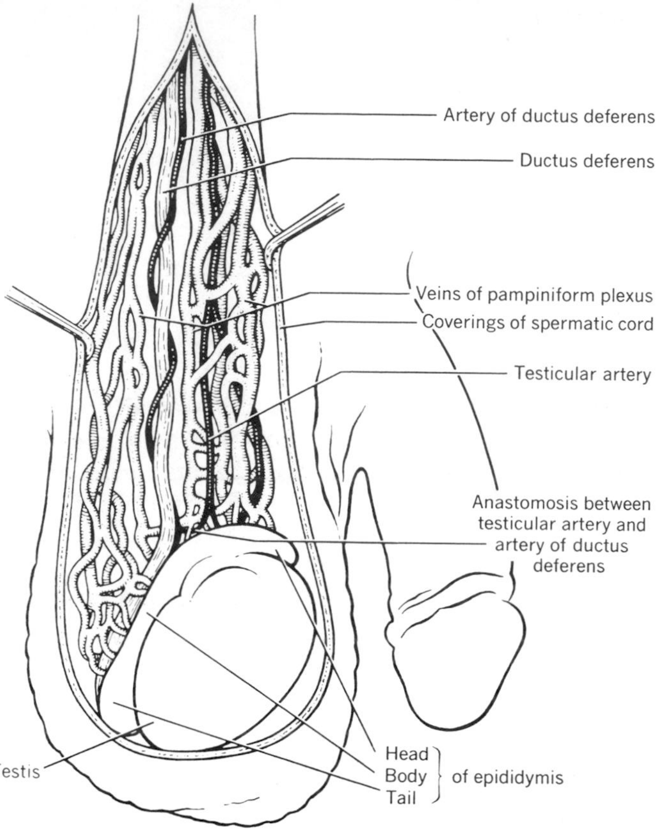

Figure 1—Dissection of right spermatic cord. The coverings of the cord have been incised and the contents separated. Notice veins of the pampiniform plexus in front and behind ductus deferens.

DISCUSSION

Applied anatomy of vasectomy

Omitting from this discussion the ethical and legal implications of vasectomy, how is this operation performed? Under local anesthesia a skin incision is made on the front of the scrotum just above the level of the head of the epididymis

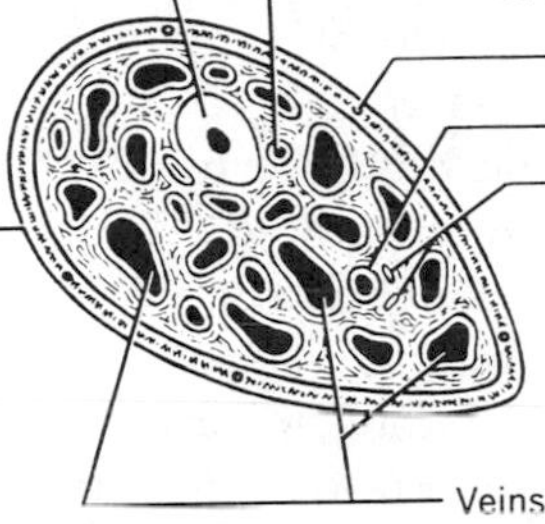

Figure 2—Cross section of spermatic cord at scrotal level of cord showing ductus deferens, veins of pampiniform plexus, testicular artery, artery of ductus deferens, and cremasteric artery.

and the ductus deferens is identified among the other constituents of the spermatic cord. What are the constituents of the spermatic cord and what are the characteristic features of the ductus deferens? The essential components of the spermatic cord are the ductus deferens with its artery, vein, and some fine nerves that pass to the epididymis, the testicular artery accompanied by testicular nerves, the pampiniform plexus of veins, lymph vessels, and the strand-like remnants of the processus vaginalis in the anterior part of the cord. All of these structures are embedded in areolar connective tissue which is in continuity with the extraperitoneal connective tissue of the abdomen (Figs. 1 and 2).

The ductus deferens lies in the posterior part of the spermatic cord and is identified by its hard and whipcord-like feel when it is rolled between the thumb and index fingers. How do you explain the firm consistency of the duct? This is due to the thick muscular wall surrounding a narrow lumen. The muscular coat consists of outer and inner longitudinal fibers and a heavy circular middle layer, and delivers by its peristaltic action the semen into the prostatic urethra during ejaculation. Is the ductus deferens the most posterior structure of the spermatic cord at the level of the incision? At this level the pampiniform (tendril-like) plexus consists of eight to ten veins, most of which lie in front of the ductus deferens. This larger anterior group surrounds the testicular artery. A smaller group, comprising two or three veins, is located posterior to the duct (Figs. 1 and 2).

In order to pick the duct for ligation the coverings of the spermatic cord are separated. What are these coverings? Although not easily identified individually, they consist of three layers, the thin internal spermatic fascia derived from the transversalis fascia, the cremasteric fascia on the outside of the former—characterized by the presence of muscular bundles of the cremaster muscle—and a thin outer covering, the external spermatic fascia, representing the continuation of the intercrural fibers of the external abdominal oblique muscle over the cord.

After the duct has been stripped free of the areolar tissue in its neighborhood, it is grasped with forceps. The small artery of the ductus deferens is either pushed aside or ligated. Of what artery is it a branch? It is derived from one of the vesical arteries, which are branches of the internal iliac artery, and accompanies the deferent duct from the pelvis through the inguinal canal as far as the testis. A small segment of the duct, 1.5 to 2 cm in length, is removed and both ends ligated. The two ends are separated and fascial tissue interposed in order to reduce the possibility of recanalization of the duct. Then the wound is closed with sutures and the operation repeated on the other side.

Does ligation of the ductus deferens lead to atrophy and nonfunctioning of the testis? Clinical and experimental evidence has shown that after ligation of the duct neither the seminiferous epithelium nor the interstitial cells degenerate. The potential for spermatogenesis is preserved after ligation. Only the ejection of spermatozoa from the testis is prevented.

What is the rationale of reunion and recanalization of the ductus deferens after previous surgical vasectomy? Can it occur spontaneously? The preservation of spermatogenesis after ligation of the duct makes it feasible to reanastomose the ligated ends in order to restore the anatomical and functional integrity of the ducts. In that case, fertility may be reestablished in 50 to 90 per cent of the operated cases.

Failure of vasectomy

Spontaneous reunion seems to take place not too infrequently, partly depending on the technique of surgery, thus defeating the purpose of ligation. The regenerated adventitia of the two ends of the duct apparently serves as a splint guiding the separated fragments to reanastomosis. What other reasons, in addition to spontaneous recanalization, could explain failure of vasectomy to result in sterility? Sperm apparently stays alive in the ampulla of the ductus deferens or in the seminal vesicle for as long as six weeks or more. During this period after ligation the patient remains, of course, potentially fertile. Another reason for failure of vasectomy is the presence of accessory ducts that bypass the ligated site. This has been reported by clinicians who reoperated such cases. Anatomists regard this as quite rare. Is the old concept that the seminal vesicles are the main storehouse for semen still tenable? The answer is negative. It is the function of the seminal vesicles to add bulk and nutritive material to the semen through its secretory activity. Live spermatozoa are stored mainly in the ductuli efferentes which connect the testis with the head of the epididymis, and in the duct of the epididymis. Nevertheless, the fact that fertile spermatozoa can be delivered for several weeks after bilateral ligation of the ductus deferens makes their storage in parts of the efferent portions of the reproductive system above the site of ligation (cranial to the epididymis) a certainty.

Other consequences of duct ligation

Is potency affected by ligation of the ducts? Potency, which is the ability of the male to have intercourse, is based on hormonal production, mainly by the testis. What cells in the testis are the source of androgen, the testicular hormone? Is the secretion of these cells interfered with by ligation? The interstitial cells of the testis which produce this hormone remain unaffected by ligation. How does this hormone leave the testis? It is secreted into the blood stream and thus potency does not suffer. Is there any justification for the opposite theory that ligation of the duct through suppression of spermatogenesis results in an increase in hormone production and therefore in improved potency? Ligation of the ductus deferens for purposes of rejuvenation and increase in masculinity was quite popular some years ago, but it is based on false claims.

Does exclusion of spermatozoa from the ejaculate after ligation make a noticeable difference in the amount of the semen? What other glands participate in the production of the ejaculate? The bulk of the semen is composed of secretions from the deferent ducts, the seminal vesicles, the prostate, and the mucous glands of the urethra, including the bulbourethral (Cowper's) glands. The amount is not much altered by the absence of spermatozoa.

Does the presence of live spermatozoa in the ejaculate a short time after ligation of the duct or after surgical reanastomosis necessarily prove fertility? There are normally approximately 300 to 500 million spermatozoa present in the semen. When the total number of sperm cells in the ejaculate falls below 70 to 150 million, sterility usually results.

Vasectomy in conjunction with prostatectomy

What other indications beside sterilization are there for ligation of the ducts? Vasectomy is commonly done preceding prostatic resection to prevent retrograde spread of infection to the epididymis. What is the channel for this spread? It travels from the prostatic urethra via the ejaculatory ducts to the ductus deferens and the epididymis. Epididymitis is a common complication of prostatectomy, the frequency of which is considerably reduced by vasectomy.

Castration by crushing of the cord

For almost fifty years a heavy clamp applied for a short time to the spermatic cord has been used by veterinarians for purposes of castration in animals. It crushes and divides the cord without breaking the skin. Recently this method has been recommended for castration purposes in patients with advanced cancer of the prostate, who might not be able to withstand open removal of the testes. The latter procedure is undertaken in order to arrest the spread of cancer by interfering with the hormonal output of the testis. Why would crushing and closed sectioning of the spermatic cord lead to castration when simple ligation of the ductus deferens does not have this effect? What is the essential difference between these two procedures? The answer lies in the interference with the blood supply to the testis taking place in the former operation, but not in the latter.

Three arteries enter into the blood supply of the testis and form an efficient anastomotic system establishing testicular circulation. Identify them and give their origin. They are, in descending order of their importance for the survival of a functioning testis, the testicular artery directly from the abdominal aorta, the artery of the ductus deferens whose origin has been given previously and which anastomoses with the testicular artery at the tail of the epididymis, and the cremasteric artery, a branch of the inferior epigastric artery. The cremasteric artery supplies the coverings of the cord and the scrotal sac and enters into functioning anastomotic connections with the testicular artery and the artery of the ductus deferens in two-thirds of all cases. All three arteries are occluded in the crushing technique described previously. What then prevents the testis from becoming necrotic in these cases where the cord is severed and the testis apparently completely deprived of its blood supply? We must assume that additional vessels that vascularize the scrotal sac, while insufficient to prevent atrophy of the testis and sterilization, assure against gangrene of the scrotal contents. They are the scrotal branches of the internal and superficial and deep external pudendal arteries.

31 Vaginismus

The following case history is taken from a note by Egerton Y. Davis in the "Correspondence" column of *Medical News*, published in 1884: [1]

> "I was sent for, about 11 PM by a gentleman whom, on my arriving at his house, I found in a state of great perturbation, and the story he told me was briefly as follows:
>
> At bedtime, when going to the back kitchen to see if the house was shut up, a noise in the coachman's room attracted his attention, and, going in he discovered to his horror that the man was in bed with one of the maids. She screamed, he struggled and they rolled out of bed together and made frantic efforts to get apart, but without success. He was a big burly man, over six feet, and she was a small woman, weighing not more than ninety pounds. She was moaning and screaming, and seemed in great agony, so that after several fruitless attempts to get them apart, he sent for me. When I arrived, I found the man standing up and supporting the woman in his arms, and it was quite evident that his penis was tightly locked in her vagina, and any attempt to dislodge it was accompanied by much pain on the part of both. It was, indeed, a case "de cohesione in coitu." I applied water, and then ice, but ineffectually, and at last sent for chloroform, a few whiffs of which sent the woman to sleep, relaxed the spasm, and relieved the captive penis, which was swollen, livid, and in a state of semi-erection, which did not go down for several hours, and for days the organ was extremely sore. The woman recovered rapidly, and seemed none the worse . . . In this case there

must have been also spasm of the muscle at the orifice, as well as higher up, for the penis seemed nipped low down, and this contraction, I think, kept the blood retained and the organ erect."

DIAGNOSIS

Vaginismus or penis captivus.

DISCUSSION

The term "vaginismus" or "vaginism" generally refers to an involuntary spasm of the vestibular opening of the vagina which prevents admission of the penis and precludes intercourse. This painful spasm of the vagina may be due to local hypersensitivity, perhaps from minor previous injuries in the vestibule, or psychologic defense mechanisms. It is characterized by involuntary contractions of various sphincters of the vagina and defense postures, such as arching of the back (lumbar lordosis) or clamping together or crossing of the thighs by the adductors. Classical anatomists were familiar with the latter fact when they designated the adductor group of the thigh as "guardian of the virgins" (custos virginum) and the first line of defense against forcible violation.

A different and very rare form of vaginismus has been reported in the literature since classical times. Here, as in our case, such severe involuntary spasm of the vaginal sphincters takes place after coital introduction of the penis that the organ cannot be withdrawn. Although reports of such occurrences have often been regarded as part of sexual folklore, they are well documented.[2–5]

Sphincters of the vagina

What are sphincters of the vagina? The beginner might be surprised by the fact that such sphincters exist at all, since in contrast to the urethra and rectum, contents of the vagina (such as menstrual blood) cannot be retained by sphincteric contraction.

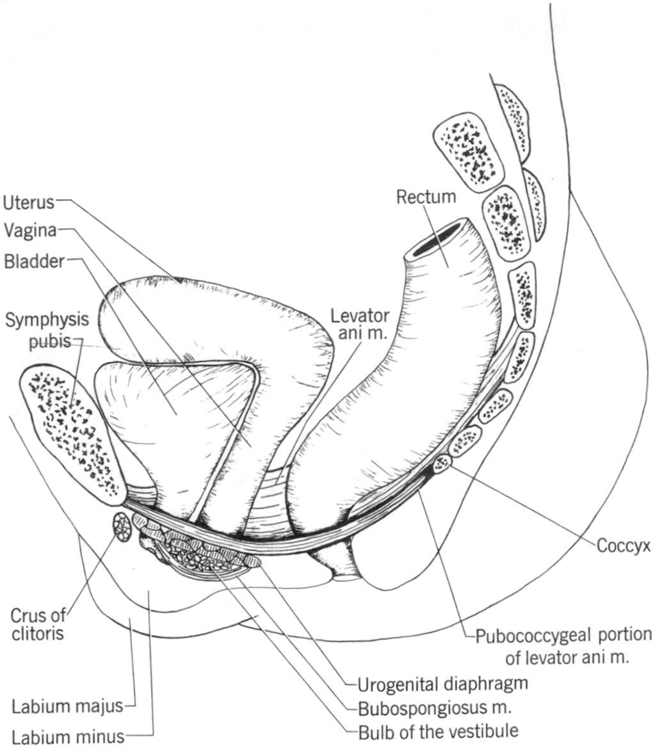

Figure 1—Parasagittal section of female pelvis, showing the three sphincters of the vagina, i.e. the bulbospongiosus, the urogenital diaphragm surrounded by its fasciae, and the pubococcygeus, a part of the levator ani. Notice the left pillar of the pubococcygeus forming part of the main sphincter of the vagina.

The externalmost sphincter of the vagina is the bulbospongiosus (bulbocavernosus). In contrast to the male, where the two halves of the muscle are united in the midline, in the female the bulbospongiosus is separated from its counterpart by the vestibule of the vagina. It arises posteriorly from the tendinous center of the perineum, the perineal body, and its fibers pass forward to surround the lowest part of the vagina. Thus, they act as weak constrictors of the vaginal orifice (Figs. 1 and 2).

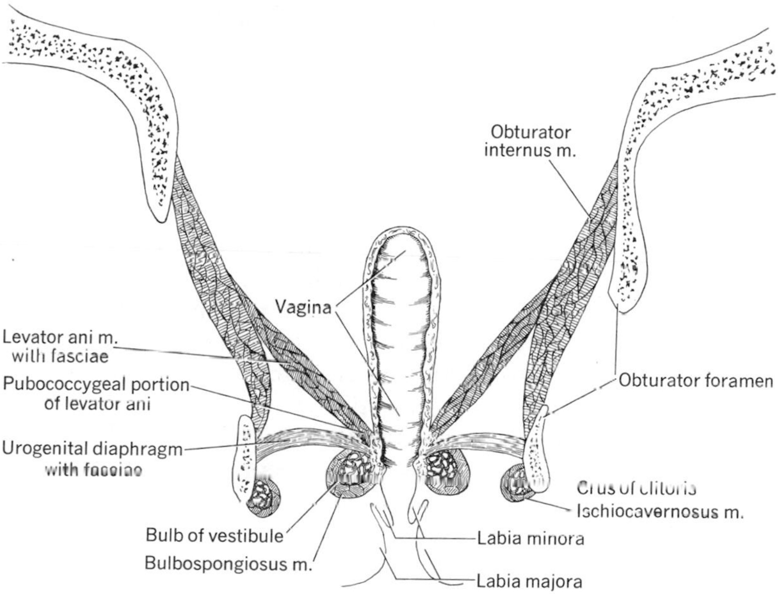

Figure 2—Coronal section of female pelvis, showing the three sphincters of the vagina, i.e., the bulbospongiosus, the urogenital diaphragm, and the pubococcygeal portion of the levator ani.

Another sphincter which surrounds the vagina at a higher level is the urogenital diaphragm. It is pierced by the urethra and vagina and is covered by membranous fasciae on its cranial and caudal aspects, the so-called superior and inferior fasciae of the urogenital diaphragm. It is less developed and more lax than in the male and extends as a thin sheet between the ischiopubic rami of the two sides. Some of its fibers surround in sphincteric fashion both the urethra and vagina, but the sphincteric portion around the urethra is stronger than that enveloping the vagina (Figs. 1 and 2).

The highest and most important sphincter of the vagina is a part of a larger muscle complex, the levator ani or pelvic diaphragm, which, hammock-like, forms the pelvic floor and separates, as a musculotendinous partition, the pelvis above from the perineum below.

Here we are concerned only with that part of the muscle which arises from the posterior aspect of the superior pubic ramus and is named the pubococcygeus. Its fibers pass around the lateral aspect of the vagina, partly to insert into it, but mostly in conjunction with its counterpart of the other side, to surround the vagina and to insert into the coccyx and the anococcygeal raphe. This portion of the levator ani is often called the constrictor vaginae (Figs. 1 and 2). Its medialmost margin can frequently be felt by vaginal examination. The normal tonus of the pubococcygeus or contraction of its inner margins narrows the vagina from side to side and is responsible for the long bars of the "H" formed on cross-section by the collapsed lumen of the vaginal tube.

One might ask to what extent the muscular layer of the vagina itself contributes to sphincteric contraction of the organ? This layer consists of poorly developed and interwoven bundles of smooth musculature with inner circular and outer longitudinal bundles. The longitudinal muscle bundles prevail. This intrinsic musculature of the vagina has no expelling or supporting functions. It serves mainly to restore the distended organ to its normal width. The question arises whether the narrowing of the vaginal tube during the sex act is not produced by the contraction of its intrinsic musculature. The answer is negative. The considerable reduction of the vaginal lumen during coitus is confined to the lower third of the vagina and is due mainly to localized congestion with maximal distention of the venus plexuses. The upper two-thirds of the vagina are actually increased in width and depth rather than contracted during the sex act.[6]

Anatomical explanation of vaginal spasm

What then is the anatomical basis for the calamitous condition in our case history which results in the embarrassing retention of the penis (known as captive penis) and which, as a number of case histories indicate, can often be resolved only by general anesthesia?

Masters and Johnson[6] in their recent monograph on the

physiologic aspects of the sex act have pointed out that in female orgasm, at the climax of the sex act, there is general increase in muscle tension accompanied by voluntary and involuntary muscle contractions. These contractions are rather widespread, involving muscles of the neck and extremities, including the gluteal musculature and the hands and feet.

At the height of the sexual response there occur involuntary rhythmic contractions of the bulbospongiosus and the lowermost portion of the vagina, as well as the muscles of the urogenital and pelvic diaphragms. Uterine contractions and spasm of the external anal and urethral sphincters have also been described.

It seems that in rare cases the involuntary muscular spasm of the pubococcygeal part of the levator ani is longer lasting, resulting in retention of the erect penis with ensuing embarrassment, which is so vividly described in our report. None of the other circularly arranged muscular structures, previously listed, such as the bulbospongiosus muscle and the urogenital diaphragm, are strong enough to bring about the retention of the male organ. Needless to say that the powerful spastic contraction of the pubococcygeus results in a vicious circle which sustains maximal erection of the penis and prevents detumescence (subsidence of erection) and withdrawal.

Frequently, analogies have been drawn between this rare form of vaginismus in the human and the familiar locking of the external sex organs in dogs. However, the underlying anatomy, particularly of the distal portion of the penis in the dog, differs to such an extent from that of the male human organ, that comparison is not helpful in explaining the human mishap.

E. Y. Davis—A pseudonym

As an appendix to this discussion, it might be interesting to return to Egerton Y. Davis, the author of the communication quoted in the beginning of this case study. His report is frequently cited as an example of this rare complication of vaginismus, particularly in textbooks of gynecology. Thus, it is the more surprising to find his name as an entry in the index to Harvey Cushing's *Life of Sir William Osler,*[7] only to be referred to the index listing: "Osler, Sir W. Personal characteristics—practical jokes." Perusal of these latter references reveals that Osler availed himself of this pseudonym for many pranks. He even signed Davis's name in hotel registers and used it as a signature for light humorous poems. As Cushing in his biography explains, one of Osler's coeditors of the *Medical News* had written a pseudo-learned editorial entitled "An Uncommon Form of Vaginismus,"[8] in which he quoted many sources back to Roman classical writers. This provoked Osler to write this imaginary case report, signing it "Egerton Y. Davis." Long before this he adopted this name as an identification of his alter ego whenever his impish nature induced him to lampoon some of his more stuffy friends and acquaintances, or even himself. Once he wrote a book review in which he pointed out an extraordinary mistake in Osler's work, and signed it, "EYD." His irrepressible spirit induced him to sign one of his last letters, written one month before his death, "EYD."

Although the colorfully written description of vaginismus by Osler utilized in our case history is fictitious, the distressing occurrence itself is quite real, particularly to the victims and may lead to serious consequences. This was true in one particular case known to the author in which the male participant committed suicide two days after the event.

REFERENCES

1. "Correspondence," *Medical News*, 45:673, 1884.
2. L. Parsons and S. C. Sommers, *Gynecology*, Philadelphia, W. B. Saunders, Co., 1962.
3. A. Benninghoff and K. Goerttler, *Lehrbuch der Anatomie des Menschen*, München-Berlin: Urban and Schwarzenberg, Vol. 2, 1964, p. 351.
4. I. Bloch, *The Sexual Life of Our Time* (translated by Dr. M. Eden Paul), New York, Falstaff Press, Inc., 1937.
5. H. Hildebrandt, "On Spasm of Levator Ani in Intercourse," Archiv f. Gynaekologie, Berlin, 1872, p. 221-232.
6. W. H. Masters and V. E. Johnson, *Human Sexual Response*, Boston: Little, Brown and Co., 1966.
7. H. Cushing, *Life of Sir William Osler*, Vols. I and II, Oxford: Clarendon Press, 1925.
8. "An Uncommon Form of Vaginismus," Medical News, 45:602-603, 1884.

Upper Extremity

32 Fracture of Clavicle

A 13-year-old boy scout fell upon his left shoulder in running down a steep incline and immediately complained of severe pain in the area of his collarbone. All movements of his left arm were painful. He tried to avoid painful motion by holding his left arm close to his body and by supporting the left elbow with his right hand.

EXAMINATION AND DIAGNOSIS

The boy is brought to a physician, who diagnoses a fracture of the clavicle. The fracture is located at the junction of the inner and middle third of the bone. There is marked tenderness and some swelling at the fracture site. Upon passing the fingers along the border of the clavicle the examiner can make out the projecting ends of the fragments. These are felt to overlap, with the sternal fragment being angulated upward and the medial end of the lateral fragment pointing backward and medially (Fig. 1). Passive movement of the left shoulder is quite painful. A roentgenogram confirms the diagnosis of clavicular fracture at the expected site and shows overriding of the fragments with depression of the outer fragment.

THERAPY AND FURTHER COURSE

The fracture is reduced by pulling the shoulder upward and backward and the correct alignment of the fragments is re-

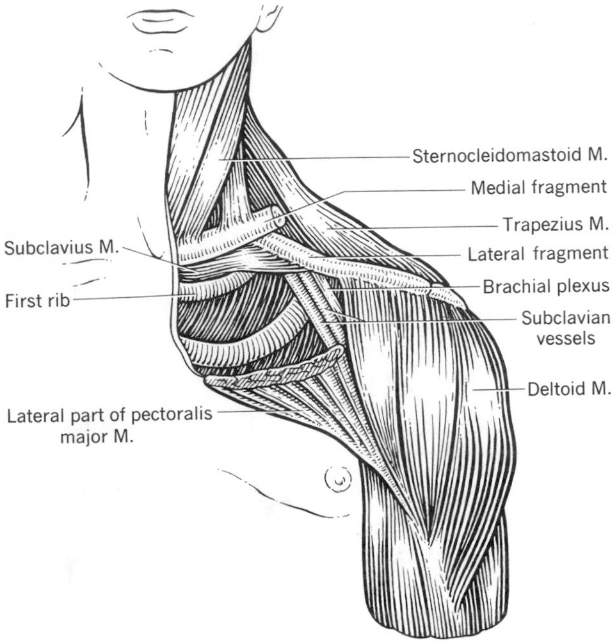

Figure 1—Fractured clavicle with typical displacement of the fragments. Notice the overriding of the fragments. Notice also how the subclavius muscle protects the underlying neurovascular structures from injury by the fragments.

tained by application of a Figure-8 bandage. This bandage allows the patient to use his left elbow, wrist, and finger joints, which are exercised at regular intervals to avoid stiffening. The bandage is removed after five weeks, when clinical examination shows evidence of bony union.

DISCUSSION

Clavicular fracture is one of the most common fractures in the body. How do you explain this? The clavicle is the only skeletal connection of the shoulder girdle to the trunk and serves as a strut to maintain the shoulder and arm at the proper distance from the chest. As such it is exposed to any force that tends to thrust the arm medially against the chest, as exemplified in our case where the patient fell on his shoulder. If unbroken, the clavicle maintains a constant distance between the acromion and the midline of the body so that a decrease in this distance, as compared with the normal side, is a rough indication of the amount of overriding of the fragments.

Ligaments anchoring the clavicle

What keeps the clavicle from dislocating in the sternoclavicular joint instead of fracturing when an inward thrust is exerted on the shoulder? Inspect a skeleton and see if there is secure adaptation of the articulating parts of this joint. As far as the bony contours are concerned, the joint seems quite unstable and vulnerable to dislocation. Why then is dislocation at this joint so infrequent? Identify the ligamentous structures that protect the integrity of the sternoclavicular joint (Fig. 2). They are the strong costoclavicular ligament, the anterior and posterior reinforcements of the articular capsule, that is, the anterior and posterior sternoclavicular ligaments, and the articular disk which is attached to the clavicle above, and the first costal cartilage below. Is there an equally strong ligament at the lateral end of the clavicle which binds the clavicle to the scapula? The coracoclavicular ligament with its two parts, the conoid and trapezoid ligaments, protects the integrity of the acromioclavicular joint and prevents the acromion from being driven under the clavicle. Can you correlate the most common site of fractures of the clavicle in the middle third with the location of the major ligaments? These fractures occur between the attachments of the ligaments that anchor the clavicle at either end, the costoclavicular and the coracoclavicular.

Clavicular fracture at birth

Do fractures of the clavicle occur as birth injuries? Fractures of the clavicle are particularly common in the newborn, in

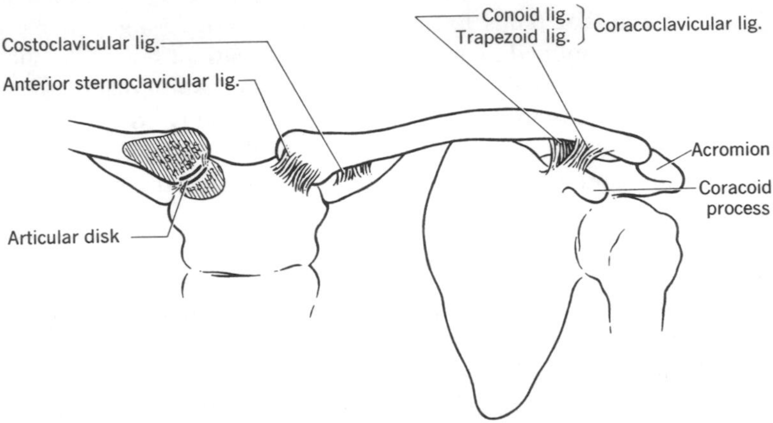

Figure 2—Ligaments of the clavicle. The disk, the sternoclavicular ligaments, and the costoclavicular ligament protect the integrity of the sternoclavicular joint and prevent dislocation. Notice that the disk is attached to the clavicle above, and the first rib below. Also notice that fractures most commonly occur between the costoclavicular and the coracoclavicular ligaments.

fact, they are more frequent than all other birth fractures combined. The clavicle may be fractured by the hand of the obstetrician in breech (buttocks) presentation or may break on its own during passage of the child through the birth canal by being pressed against the maternal symphysis pubis. Can you give a reason why the clavicle at the time of birth would be well ossified and therefore rather rigid and unyielding? The clavicle starts its ossification earlier than any other bone, i.e. during the fifth week of fetal life.

Muscles involved in clavicular fracture

The displacement of the fragments is rather characteristic and depends on the action of the muscles attached to the shoulder girdle and on the weight of the arm. The pull of what muscle displaces the medial fragment upward? The clavicular portion of the sternocleidomastoid muscle is responsible for the upward tilt of this fragment (Fig. 1).

On the other hand, the weight of the arm and the pull of what muscle would displace the lateral fragment downward? The deltoid arises from the lateral third of the clavicle and combined with the weight of the arm is responsible for this displacement. These factors cause the left arm to hang lower than the right. What large muscle connecting the thorax with the arm would adduct, that is, pull the arm toward the thorax, causing a decrease in the distance between acromion and midline and therefore an overlapping of the fragments? The pectoralis major, supported by the latissimus dorsi and smaller muscles, is responsible for this displacement. Since the medial rotators of the arm are stronger than the lateral, and the bracing action of the clavicle is nullified by the fracture, the arm is also medially rotated. What are the muscles responsible for this action? The pectoralis major, the subscapularis, the teres major, and the latissimus dorsi are the medial rotators of the arm. This medial rotation of the arm also explains why the medial end of the lateral fragment points posteriorly.

In spite of the superficial location of the clavicle and the frequent presence of bony fragments at the site of fracture, piercing of the skin by osseous spicules is rather rare. Can you give any reason for this? The subcutaneous location of the platysma, which allows the skin to move freely over the clavicle, protects the skin and usually prevents fragments from piercing it, thus preventing the occurrence of a compound (open) fracture with its dangers of secondary infection at the fracture site.

More important even is the protective action of another muscle that lies deep to the clavicle, between it and the first rib, and guards important underlying structures against injuries from bony fragments. Name this muscle and the underlying structures. The subclavius surrounded by its fascial sheath, derived from the clavipectoral fascia, runs from the first rib to the undersurface of the clavicle and shields the subclavian vessels and the brachial plexus from damage in clavicular fracture. Remember that these important structures pass over the first rib but under the clavicle on their way into the axilla. Do the curvatures of the clavicle make allowance for the course of these neurovascular structures? The medial half of the clavicle has its convexity anteriorly, thus increasing the space between it and the first rib. It might help you, however, to visualize the crowding of the subclavian vessels in the costoclavicular space if you know that in many people the radial pulse becomes demonstrably weaker if you pull the arm forcibly in a posterior and downward direction.

Injuries to blood vessels and nerves in clavicular fracture

Watson-Jones in his textbook, entitled *Fractures and Joint Injuries*, tells us that the founder of the London police force, Sir Robert Peel, (from whom the members of this force derive their nickname "bobby") died of a fractured clavicle, with splinters from the fractured bone causing a fatal hemorrhage from the subclavian vein. Other cases are on record where non-union of the clavicular fracture or excessive callus formation was responsible for thrombosis of either the subclavian vein or artery, causing pulmonary embolism in the former and embolism to the brachial or basilar arteries in the latter. Describe the course that a blood clot has to take to reach the lung in the case of venous thrombosis and to lodge in the basilar artery in thrombosis of the subclavian artery. Brachiocephalic vein, superior vena cava, right atrium, right ventricle, and pulmonary artery would be the pathway that a blood clot formed in the subclavian vein would take on its way to the lung. A blood clot formed in the subclavian artery would travel with the arterial bloodstream to the periphery of the upper extremity, where it would be arrested in one of the major arteries of the extremity, depending on the size of the clot. It also could go up to the brain via the vertebral branch of the subclavian artery and the basilar artery at the base of the brain.

Injuries to the brachial plexus have likewise been described as early or late complications of clavicular fracture. The neurologic symptoms consist of paresthesias (sensations of tingling, burning, and numbness) in the area of distribution of segments C8 and T1. Which trunk of the brachial plexus is involved? The lower trunk and particularly its first thoracic component lies behind the subclavian artery on the first rib and is exposed to pressure against the rigid bone.

From the anatomical point it is quite interesting to note that a nerve, which occasionally runs through a foramen in the clavicle, may be embedded in the callus and pressed upon, thus causing severe pain following a clavicular fracture. What is this nerve that may normally pierce the bone? It is a branch of the middle supraclavicular nerve which may have to be resected in these cases.

33 Cervical Rib

A widow, 39, has suffered for many years from "rheumatic" pains in her right arm. Recently, after taking on additional housework, the pain has worsened and radiates down the medial side of arm and forearm into the hand. Sometimes the fingers on the ulnar side of the hand tingle and feel numb. The right arm seems to be weaker than the left.

EXAMINATION

Examination shows some tenderness and resistance in the right supraclavicular area, but nothing definite can be palpated. Downward pulling on the arm increases the pain. There is obvious wasting of the right thenar eminence. On testing, the opponens pollicis and abductor pollicis brevis seem to be particularly involved.

DIAGNOSIS

The diagnosis of cervical rib in this case is based on the resistance in the right supraclavicular fossa and on the presence of subjective and objective neurologic signs pointing to involvement of the lower trunk of the brachial plexus, with both sensory and motor fibers being affected. The roentgenogram confirms the diagnosis and shows an accessory rib on the right side articulating with the seventh cervical vertebra, pointing forward and downward and ending bluntly.

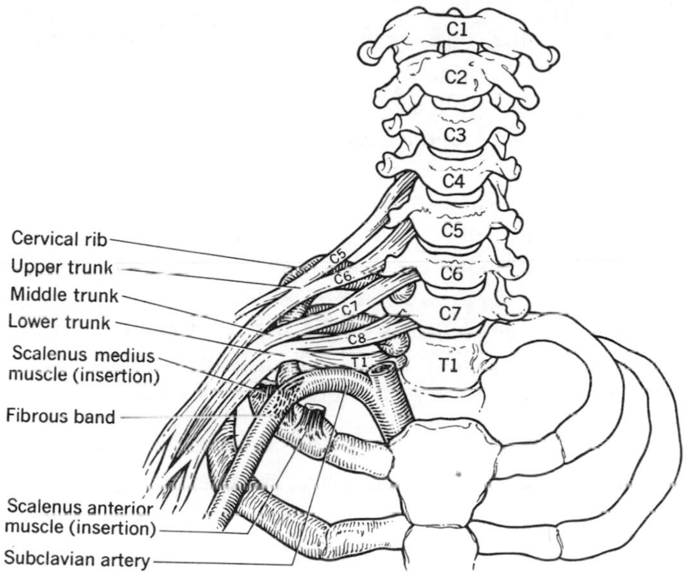

Figure 1—Cervical rib on the right side is continued as fibrous band which attaches to first rib. Brachial plexus and subclavian artery are elevated and lowest trunk of brachial plexus seems particularly taut and stretched by cervical rib.

THERAPY

At operation the cervical rib was found to be continued anteriorly as a fibrous band which was attached to the first rib. The brachial plexus was elevated as was also the subclavian artery. Both were seen passing over the cervical rib. The lowest trunk of the plexus appeared rather taut and stretched over the accessory rib (Fig. 1). The cervical rib was excised.

FURTHER COURSE

After removal of the cervical rib the symptoms gradually disappeared during the next few months. Strength seemed to come back to the hand and the wasting of the thenar eminence also gradually diminished.

DISCUSSION

The sensory disturbances in this case do not correspond to the cutaneous distribution of any one peripheral nerve, but involve an area that is supplied by at least three named nerves. Which are these? The medial brachial and antebrachial cutaneous nerves and the ulnar nerve supply the involved area with sensory fibers. In addition the motor defect in the thenar eminence concerns two muscles supplied by a fourth nerve (name it), and not at all the muscles supplied by the ulnar nerve, whose fibers are mainly involved on the sensory side. The two affected muscles of the thenar compartment are supplied by the median nerve. The involvement of fibers distributed through four peripheral nerves makes highly improbable a peripheral nerve lesion, such as paralysis of the median or ulnar nerves.

Localization of neural lesion

A lesion involving sensory and motor nerve fibers, proximal to the level at which the nerves of distribution of the brachial plexus are formed, would explain all sensory and motor defects in this case.

Using a dermatome chart (Fig. 2), state which neural segments are involved on the sensory side. C8 and T1 are the segments affected on the sensory side. Statements in several anatomical texts notwithstanding, the weight of neurological evidence indicates that the two muscles involved, that is, the opponens pollicis and the abductor pollicis brevis, most commonly receive their main motor supply via the median nerve from segments C8 and T1. These are the same segments that display the sensory defects.

It is most likely that the lesion is located outside the cord distal to the point where sensory and motor fibers combine to form the mixed spinal nerve, since both types of fibers are involved. The lesion actually must be beyond the point of division of the mixed spinal nerve into ventral and dorsal primary rami, since there is no sign of neurological deficiency in the dorsal primary rami of C8 and T1.

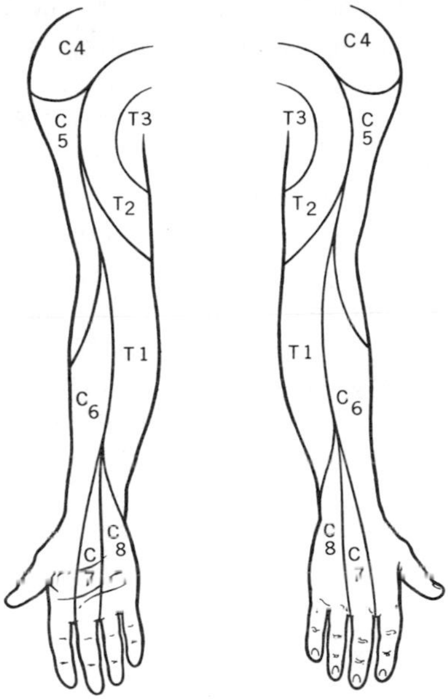

Figure 2—Dermatome chart of anterior and posterior aspects of upper extremity (after Foerster). Note particularly representation of segments C8 and T1 on medial side of arm, forearm, and hand.

How many ventral primary rami are affected? Where in the course of the ventral primary rami of C8 and T1 did the lesion most likely occur? The pathological picture as displayed at operation reveals that it is the lower trunk of the brachial plexus that is exposed to the stretching effect of the accessory rib. All clinical signs also point to the lower trunk of the brachial plexus as the site of the lesion. This would explain all subjective and objective neurologic disturbances including the motor deficiencies.

Clinical examination shows that in our case the opponens pollicis and the abductor pollicis brevis are particularly involved. How would you test the action of these muscles? Keep in mind that it is the function of the abductor pollicis to pull the thumb away from the palm in a plane at right angles to the palm and of the opponens pollicis to advance the thumb across the palm in an arc, rotating it simultaneously, so that at the end of the motion the palmar surfaces of the thumb and little finger are in opposition to each other. Consequently you test these muscles for integrity of function by letting them execute these motions against resistance.

Further clinical study reveals that certainly not all motor fibers coming from C8 and T1 are affected, for example, the muscles of the hypothenar eminence seem to have escaped. This is common in nerve lesions and probably can be explained on the basis of the location of nerve fibers within the trunk and perhaps also on the basis of special susceptibility of certain fibers to pressure.

34 Embolism of Brachial Artery

Mr. F. H., aged 51, is admitted to the hospital for generalized arteriosclerosis, lesions of the aortic valves, and cardiac failure. During his stay in the hospital, he suddenly complains of sharp pain and partial paralysis of the right forearm of about one hour's duration.

EXAMINATION

On examination the forearm is cold and pale, with the hand and fingers drawn up in a contracted position. There is loss of motor power and sensation below the elbow. Radial and ulnar pulsations are absent.

DIAGNOSIS

Embolism of the brachial artery, that is, occlusion of the artery by a blood clot originating elsewhere in the bloodstream.

THERAPY

The patient is taken to surgery, where a long incision is made over the brachial artery in the medial bicipital groove. The median nerve is dissected free and retracted out of the way. The incision is extended into the cubital fossa and the bicipital

The case history is taken from a paper by R. D. Duncan and M. E. Myers, entitled "Peripheral Arterial Embolism. Brachial Embolism Successfully Treated," Am. J. Surg., 62:34 (Oct.) 1943.

aponeurosis (lacertus fibrosus) is cut, thus exposing the bifurcation of the brachial artery.

On exposing the brachial artery the clot within the vessel can be seen easily. The clot completely fills the brachial artery and extends about one inch into the radial and ulnar arteries. The entire brachial artery is occluded as well as the deep brachial and all of the collateral branches, including the radial and ulnar recurrent vessels. Rubber bands are placed above and below the embolus. A small incision one inch long is made just above the bifurcation of the brachial artery, and the extensions of the clot into the radial and ulnar arteries are removed with forceps. The remainder of the clot in the brachial artery is removed by a combination of suction and milking. A small, soft rubber catheter lubricated with vaseline is introduced into the artery as a means of suction, and the milking action is carried out manually. The small arterial incision is then closed with sutures. The clot at operation measures eight inches in length and completely occludes the collateral arterial vessels. Amputation would certainly have been required if the patient had not been operated.

FURTHER COURSE

Immediately postoperatively, the radial pulse at the wrist could easily be felt. Motor power and sensation in the forearm and hand gradually returned to normal and four days later the patient was seen using his right hand to feed himself. He was discharged from the hospital.

The patient did not receive anticoagulants since this history antedates the advent of these drugs.

DISCUSSION

The diagnosis of occlusion of the brachial artery by a blood clot originating elsewhere in the bloodstream, was based on the appearance of sudden sharp pain, on the loss of motor power and sensory function, on the coolness and paleness of the extremity, and on the absence of pulsations. All this took place in an individual suffering from chronic heart and aortic disease, which is conducive to the formation of thrombi in the heart and aorta. The signs listed are typical of arterial embolism, that is, the spread of a blood clot, which in this case was formed in a diseased heart or aorta. Give the course of such a clot from the left ventricle to the right brachial artery. The clot traveled from the left ventricle to the ascending aorta where, at the beginning of the aortic arch, it passed into the brachiocephalic trunk, from there into the right subclavian and axillary arteries, and then into the brachial artery where it was arrested.

Location of pulse in ulnar and radial arteries

Both ulnar and radial pulsations were absent. Where would you try to find the pulse of either artery? Remember that the pulse is best felt in areas where the artery is superficial and resting on a firm structure such as a bone or a dense ligament. This is the case for both arteries at the wrist where the ulnar artery lies superficial to the flexor retinaculum on the radial side of the pisiform bone and ulnar nerve. The pulse of the radial artery is felt on the lateral side of the wrist a little more proximally, lateral to the tendon of the flexor carpi radialis.

What is the cause of the partial motor paralysis and the loss of sensation? Remember that nerves and muscles can function only in the presence of sufficient blood supply, which was interrupted in our case by the arterial embolus (clot).

Surgically important relations of the brachial artery

During surgery the median nerve had to be identified and retracted. What is its changing relationship to the brachial artery? The median nerve in the arm usually crosses in front of, rarely behind, the brachial artery from lateral above to medial below. In the cubital fossa the median nerve is medial to the brachial artery (Fig. 1). Beginners often mistake the basilic vein and the medial cutaneous nerve of the forearm for the brachial artery and the median nerve. What separates the

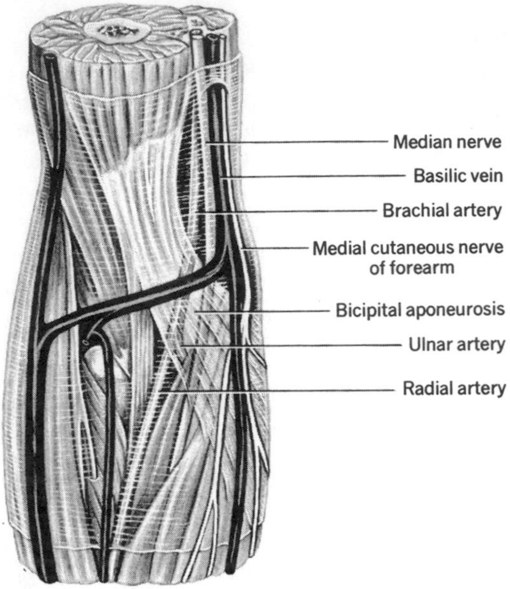

Figure 1—Structures along the medial aspect of the cubital fossa.

brachial artery from the basilic vein in the lower part of the arm? The deep (antebrachial) fascia and the bicipital aponeurosis separate the brachial artery from the more superficially located vein (Fig. 1). Remember also that the brachial artery usually is accompanied by two veins.

What is the surgical landmark for the level of the bifurcation of the brachial artery? The neck of the radius is generally given as the usual level, but the bifurcation may be located more proximally.

Collateral circulation in blockage of the brachial artery

Surprising, at the time of surgery, was the large size of the clot which not only occluded the brachial artery, but also its most important branches, the deep brachial and the two terminal branches, the radial and ulnar arteries. The collateral branches around the elbow were likewise occluded. Undoubtedly the large extent of the clot was due to secondary thrombosis above and below the embolus. There was, therefore, in this case no chance for the development of a collateral circulation, but in milder cases the limb may survive without specific treatment due to the anastomosing channels around the site of the obstruction.

In case of non-intervention, survival of the limb depends on the presence of anastomosing channels which bypass the site of blockage to transport blood to the periphery around the occlusion. What are the anastomosing channels if the block in the brachial artery is above the origin of the deep brachial artery? This is a most unfavorable site and the circulation relies essentially on the anastomosis between the descending branch of the posterior humeral circumflex artery from the axillary, and an ascending branch of the deep brachial artery.

A block below the origin of the deep brachial artery is more favorable. Here numerous anastomosing vessels are available above and below the block to re-establish the circulation. It is probably not necessary to familiarize oneself with the names of all of these vessels, if one realizes that the deep brachial divides into anterior and posterior descending branches and the brachial artery itself sends distally the superior and inferior ulnar collateral arteries. These descending vessels, which all have "collateral" in their name, anastomose with "recurrent" branches from the radial, the ulnar, and the dorsal interosseous artery in front of and behind the elbow. Cross-anastomoses from the radial to the ulnar side likewise exist. In addition there are many unnamed vascular channels available, particularly those present in the musculature.

As stated before, in our case the blockage was so extensive that a collateral circulation could not be established. But for the operation the limb would have had to be sacrificed.

35 Intravenous Injection

Mrs. C. F., a 42-year-old housewife, came to the hospital with a history of heart disease following repeated attacks of rheumatic fever. At present the patient complains of cough and severe shortness of breath and swelling of her legs.

EXAMINATION

On examination the patient appears in acute distress from shortness of breath. The heart is considerably enlarged; there is fluid in the pleural cavity; the liver is increased in size. There is marked edema of the legs, particularly in the region of the ankles. The roentgenogram shows signs of pulmonary congestion with fluid in the pleural cavity.

DIAGNOSIS

The diagnosis is heart failure resulting from a rheumatic heart lesion.

THERAPY AND FURTHER COURSE

The patient was put immediately on sedatives, cardiac medication, and mercurial diuretics. For the first few days of treatment the intravenous route (I.V.) was chosen in order to accelerate the diuretic effect.

While the first three injections into the cubital veins were painless and well tolerated, on the fourth injection the patient complained immediately of burning pain at the site of injection in a vein in the lateral portion of the cubital fossa. The pain increased during the day and radiated over the volar aspect of the forearm. In the evening, the patient complained of numbness and prickling over the radial aspect of the forearm. Intravenous medication was continued in the other arm.

Under prescribed treatment the patient improved gradually and was discharged for ambulatory treatment. However, the numbness over the lateral part of the forearm persisted. Palpation of the cubital fossa showed an indurated area at the previous site of the painful injection. There is no muscular atrophy and motion of the forearm and hand is normal. However, there is complete loss for all modalities of sensation over most of the area of the lateral antebrachial cutaneous nerve.

DISCUSSION

What is the rationale of intravenous medication? The intravenous route is chosen when a rapid effect is needed and application directly into the bloodstream appears indicated. What is the favorite site for I.V. injections and why is this location chosen?

Applied anatomy of the cubital and antebrachial veins

The median cubital vein is most frequently utilized for venipuncture (taking of a blood sample), venesection (blood letting), intravenous injection of drugs, and blood transfusions because the vein is large, superficially located, and therefore easily seen and felt. It is also unaccompanied by nerves and arteries. Which two superficial veins does the median cubital vein connect? In the most common type of arrangement the cephalic and basilic veins on the lateral and medial sides of the forearm are joined by the median cubital vein which crosses the roof of the cubital fossa in a medially ascending direction (Fig. 1). The vein which is present in about three-fourths of

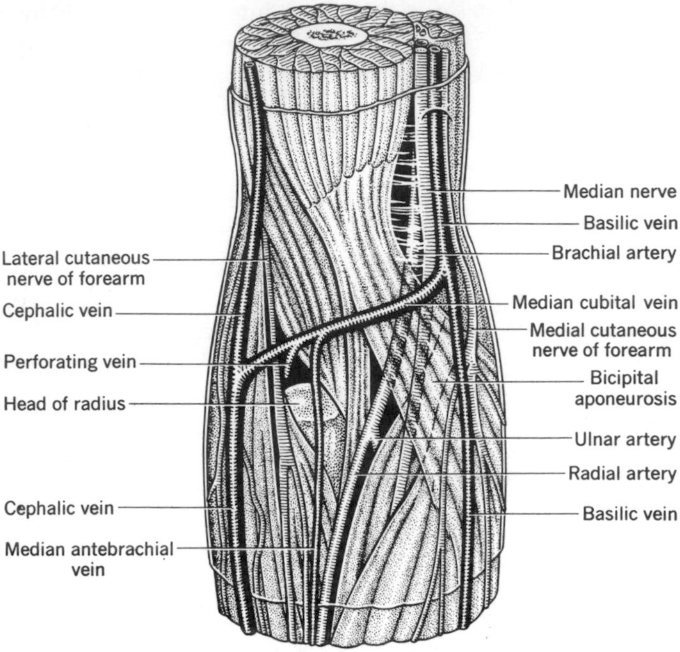

Figure 1—Superficial veins of elbow and forearm mostly accompanied by cutaneous nerves. Note the relationship of basilic vein to median nerve and brachial artery. Notice that the median cubital vein is unaccompanied by nerves. Notice, also, its deep connection by a perforating vein.

all cases terminates in the basilic vein by ascending along the medial margin of the biceps muscle.

Do other superficial veins likewise connect with the median cubital vein? It frequently also receives blood from the median antebrachial vein which ascends on the volar aspect of the forearm about halfway between the cephalic and basilic veins. Quite frequently the median antebrachial vein bifurcates at the elbow into two veins, with one of these joining the cephalic vein and the other the basilic (Fig. 2). Thus, an M-shaped arrangement results. The two central limbs of the M are then frequently spoken of as the median cephalic and median

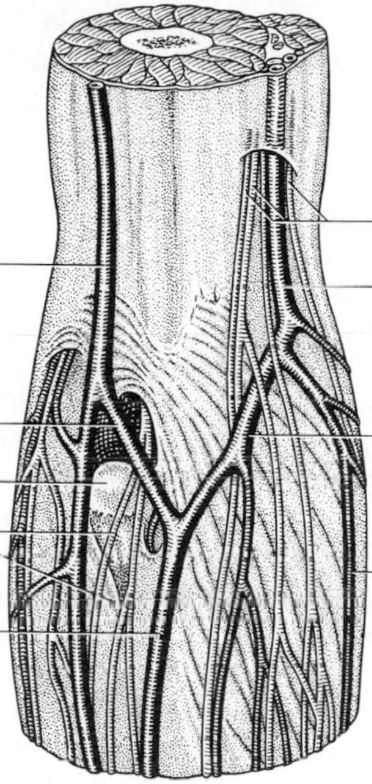

Figure 2—The M-shaped arrangement of cubital veins.

basilic veins, the latter corresponding to the previously mentioned median cubital vein. Does this vein drain exclusively into the cephalic and basilic veins? There exists in addition a communication with the deep veins of the forearm which passes through an opening in the deep fascia (Fig. 1).

How do you increase the state of distention of the superficial veins for the purpose of venipuncture? The following means are customarily employed: (1) Keeping the arm in a dependent position for some time which slows the venous return. (2) Compression of the veins by a tourniquet 1.5 to 2 in. above the site of the puncture. (3) Application of heat by means of hot, moist towels or by immersing the hand and forearm into a basin of hot water. (4) Alternating opening and closing of the hand. What is the effect of the latter procedure and what is the result if the tourniquet is applied too tightly? Muscular activity will increase the amount of arterial blood flow to the distal portion of the extremity. It is also possible that the opening and closing of the hand will enhance the blood flow from the deep to the superficial veins by means of the perforating veins. On the other hand, maximum tightening of the tourniquet may obstruct the arterial flow to the forearm.

Thrombosis formation with occlusion of the injected vein is a frequent consequence of I.V. injection. This obliteration of the vein may be asymptomatic or it may transform the vein through the accompanying inflammatory process into a knotty cord, which may remain painful and tender for many months. The obliteration of the vein can be caused by the simple trauma of venipuncture or more frequently as a direct result of the irritating effect of the injected drug. It then becomes necessary, as in our case, to inject other veins in the cubital region or in the forearm. The cephalic, basilic, and median antebrachial veins are available. What are the risks of utilizing any of these veins? In contrast to the median cubital vein, these veins are accompanied by cutaneous nerves which may be injured (Fig. 1).

Nerve injuries by intravenous injection

In case of leakage of the injected drug from the vein after withdrawal of the needle or through faulty extravenous injection of part of the drug, some nerves may readily be damaged. Identify them. They are the lateral antebrachial cutaneous nerve, whose branches course with the cephalic and median antebrachial veins; and the medial antebrachial cutaneous nerve, which accompanies the basilic vein. What is the origin of these two nerves and what cutaneous area do they supply? The lateral antebrachial cutaneous nerve is the terminal cutaneous branch of the musculocutaneous nerve. It pierces the deep fascia lateral to the biceps above the elbow joint and divides into anterior and posterior branches to supply the front and back of the radial side of the forearm. It may also supply a variable area of skin on the dorsum of the hand. By contrast, the medial antebrachial cutaneous nerve is a direct branch of the medial cord of the brachial plexus. It pierces the deep fascia medial to the biceps at the middle of the arm, and dividing into anterior and ulnar branches, supplies the skin on the front and back of the ulnar side of the forearm. What nerve was involved in our case? The injection injured the anterior branch of the lateral antebrachial cutaneous nerve.

What precautions should be taken to prevent extravenous injection of medication? The gauge of the needle should be as small as possible, the needle should be sharp, the skin over the site of the injection tightened, and the piston of the syringe aspirated to verify location of the needle in the vein. Finally, the injection should be done slowly to prevent leakage during injection and after withdrawal of the needle. Which is the important motor nerve that is exposed to damage by I.V. injection in this area (Fig. 1)? Injury to the median nerve, often in combination with impairment of the medial antebrachial cutaneous nerve, has been described. The result is severe loss of motor function in the muscles supplied by the median nerve and sensory deficiencies in the territory of the median and medial antebrachial cutaneous nerves. For this reason it has been recommended not to give any injections in the basilic vein above the bend of the elbow.

Inadvertent intra-arterial injection

Another complication, likewise quite serious, is accidental intra-arterial injection. What artery may be involved and what separates this artery from the basilic vein (Fig. 1)? If one realizes that only the deep fascia and the bicipital aponeurosis separate the basilic vein from the brachial artery, one understands that such accidents occur not too infrequently and are perhaps sometimes well tolerated. What clue would you have that the needle was in the brachial artery instead of in a vein? The aspirated blood would be bright red and not dark red, but this criterion could be nullified if the needle at first entered the vein and only in the course of the injection pierced the venous wall and slipped into the artery. In the case of irritating drugs, the clinical picture of arterial or para-arterial injection is ushered in by the occurrence of severe burning pain in the hand and forearm. This is followed by dead-white blanching of the hand and distal portions of the forearm and disappearance of the radial pulse. The outcome is frequently gangrene of the fingers and distal portions of the forearm, necessitating amputation. The underlying pathology is early or late thrombosis of the brachial artery or one or both of its terminal branches, combined with distal arterial and arteriolar spasm. How do you explain the immediate maximal arterial constriction that is noted in these cases? This is due to intense spasm of the smooth muscle of the arterial wall as result of the irritation and injury to the vessel. Reflex contraction of the vascular wall following stimulation of the sympathetic vascular plexus may also be a reason. Blockage of the vasa vasorum by the contraction of their muscular wall may contribute to the damage of the intima, enhancing the vascular thrombosis.

Can you name one arterial anomaly which would make intra-arterial injection more likely to occur? A superficial ulnar artery may arise from the brachial artery high in the arm, to course down the forearm superficial to the volar muscles and either superficial or deep to the deep fascia. It occurs in approximately 3 to 6 per cent of all cases and is apt to be mistaken for a vein for purposes of injection or may be injured accidentally when the accompanying basilic vein is injected. If, in the course of I.V. anesthesia, the superficial ulnar artery is injected erroneously, death may result. Will the anesthesia after intra-arterial injection occur earlier or later than after I.V. application? The agent injected into the arterial bloodstream will not immediately reach the heart and brain, but pass through the capillary system first and it will be diluted. Thus, intra-arterial anesthesia occurs later and a fatal overdose may be given.

Venous embolism

Contrary to expectation, dislodgement of a blood clot (embolism) from a vein that has been thrombosed by frequent injection, takes place only exceptionally. Can you give an explanation for this fact? The thrombi in the damaged vein are so firmly anchored by the concomitant inflammation that displacement via the venous bloodstream is very rare.

On the other hand, inadvertent introduction of an air embolus into the venous circulation during I.V. injections and transfusions is a recognized danger of which one has to be aware. In taking blood from donors, collection bottles may develop positive air pressure creating conditions for air embolism with resulting serious cardiac and pulmonary complications. Review the pathway of such an air embolus from the median cubital vein to the pulmonary artery. It would go by way of the median cubital into the basilic, the axillary, the subclavian, the brachiocephalic vein, the superior vena cava, the right atrium and ventricle, and into the pulmonary artery. In a heroic self-experiment one investigator injected himself with 5 to 10 cc. of air intravenously which led only to a quickly passing sensation of oppression in the cardiac area. In what veins would the danger of air embolism be greater? The large veins of the neck and the axillary area are predisposed to air embolism by puncture due to the negative pressure in their lumen and the fascial attachment to their wall which prevents them from collapsing when opened.

Other veins utilized for intravenous injection

Name other superficial veins that are suitable for puncture and injection, in case the cubital veins and veins of the forearm are too small or are obliterated after frequent injections. Difficulties in the selection of an adequate vein arise particularly in small infants, if large quantities of fluid, plasma, or blood have to be given. The following veins can be utilized: metacarpal and metatarsal veins and the veins of the dorsal venous arch of the hand and foot; the greater saphenous vein in the ankle; the greater and lesser saphenous veins in the leg; the femoral and greater saphenous veins in the thigh; the veins of the scalp and the external jugular vein. In rare cases in the infant the venous sinuses of the skull have been utilized by puncturing them through the open fontanelles. If the femoral and greater saphenous veins in the thigh and the latter vein in the ankle are used for transfusions, particularly in infants, they are dissected out under local anesthesia in a "cut-down" procedure and a catheter may be passed into them. What is the relation of the greater saphenous vein to the malleolus of the ankle and the medial condyle of the tibia? It runs in front of the medial malleolus where it can easily be seen and felt but posterior to the medial condyle of the tibia.

36 Tendon Sheath and Thenar Space Infections

Ten days before coming to the hospital the patient cut his right index finger just above the metacarpophalangeal joint on a tin can. The wound became infected and the patient consulted a physician who opened the wound and passed a drainage tube through and across the dorsum coming out between index and middle finger on the dorsum of the hand.

EXAMINATION

Upon examination the index finger is seen to be much swollen, as is the entire hand, particularly the dorsum. Several openings appear about the proximal phalanx of the index finger. On probing one of these openings, it is found to communicate with the metacarpophalangeal joint of the index finger. The entire finger and hand are slightly tender, but marked and conspicuous tenderness is elicited over the flexor tendon sheath of the index finger and is sharply circumscribed over it, being most acute at its proximal end over the metacarpophalangeal articulation. Flexion of the index finger does not increase pain; but extension causes marked pain throughout the finger. The pain is most sharply noted by the patient at the proximal end of the tendon sheath. Extension of other fingers causes little increase of pain. There is no particular pain on the dorsum of the index finger where the cuts are found. Axillary lymph

Based upon actual case history taken from A. B. Kanavel's Infections of the Hand, **sixth edition, Lea and Febiger, Philadelphia, 1933.**

nodes on the diseased side are markedly swollen. The patient has a temperature of 101° and acceleration of pulse.

Although the swelling is most noticeable over the dorsum of the hand, it should be realized as an important principle of all hand infections that the site of greatest swelling does not necessarily indicate the location of pus collection.

DIAGNOSIS

Infected wound of index finger, tendon sheath infection of flexor sheath of index finger, involvement of metacarpophalangeal joint, lymph vessel and lymph node infection.*

THERAPY AND FURTHER COURSE

The flexor tendon sheath over the index finger is opened from end to end and pus evacuated. The dorsal openings are also enlarged. Hot dressings are applied. The temperature continues to run between 99° and 101°. Ten days later there is marked ballooning in the thenar area with tenderness localized in this area. The patient is reoperated and the thenar space drained from the dorsum. A drainage tube from the space to the dorsum is inserted. The infection continues and leads to destruction of the metacarpophalangeal joint and the proximal phalanx of the index finger. A month later, after amputation of the index finger including the head of the second metacarpal, the patient improves rapidly and is discharged from the hospital. He has good function of thumb and remaining fingers.

DISCUSSION

We are dealing here with a progressive infection of the hand, which started from a minor injury but lead to a serious infection of the flexor tendon sheath of the index finger with involve-

* For a concise but somewhat schematic anatomical discussion of the tendon sheaths and deep spaces in the palm of the hand the student is referred to A. L. McGregor's A Synopsis of Surgical Anatomy, tenth edition, Williams and Wilkins, Baltimore, 1969, pp. 257-60 and pp. 671-76.

ment of the bones and the metacarpophalangeal joint of that finger and secondary spread to the thenar space. Another complication was the lymph vessel and lymph node infection that accompanied the local spread.

Nowadays application of antibiotics might have mitigated the progressive course of this infection, although surgical intervention is usually necessary to stop the spread of the infection.

Infection of tendon sheath

The marked and conspicuous tenderness over the tendon sheath of the index finger establishes the diagnosis of tendon sheath infection. What tendons are located in this tendon sheath? The tendons to the index finger from the flexor digitorum superficialis and profundus are within this tendon sheath. Where does this tendon sheath end proximally, and where distally? The sheath ends proximally at the neck of the second metacarpal and distally at the base of the third phalanx (Fig. 1). Why is extension of the involved finger so painful as compared with flexion? It puts the involved tendons and their sheath on the stretch.

Infection of thenar space

The ballooning of the thenar region with tenderness over it is a typical sign of thenar space infection. Spread of infection from the proximal end of the tendon sheaths of the fingers to the deep spaces in the palm of the hand is quite common because the digital flexor sheaths of the second, third, and fourth fingers begin at the level where the deep spaces end (Fig. 1). Where is this level? It is approximately at the level of the distal palmar crease.

Which are the deep spaces in the palm of the hand that frequently harbor and confine infections? The midpalmar space medially and the thenar space laterally are the spaces that lie deep to the flexor tendons in the palm. They are sometimes also called the medial and lateral deep palmar spaces. Infection of

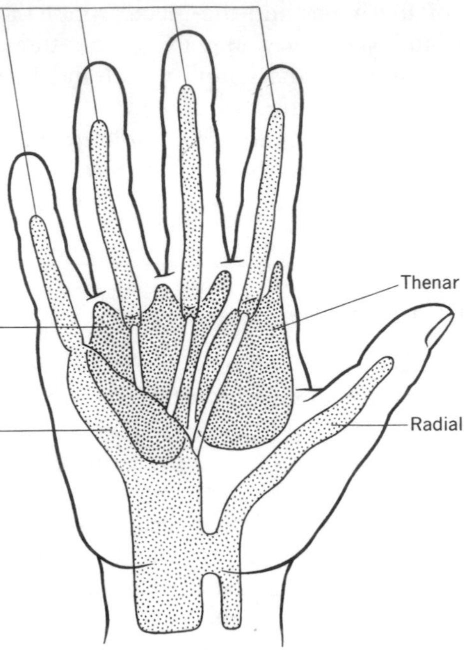

Figure 1—Shows the radial and ulnar bursae and the flexor tendon sheaths of the second, third, and fourth fingers as well as the deep spaces in the palm of the hand. Notice how infection of the tendon sheath of the index finger could easily involve the thenar space.

which tendon sheath may lead most commonly to involvement of the thenar space, as in this case? Infection of the tendon sheath of the index finger may rupture into the thenar space. Infection of the tendon sheath of the flexor pollicis longus (the radial bursa) may likewise perforate into the thenar space. The reverse may happen with a primary infection of the thenar space breaking into the radial bursa (Fig. 1). What are the superficial, deep, lateral, and medial boundaries of the thenar space? The thenar space is bounded superficially by the tendons of the index and sometimes also of the middle finger; its deep boundary is the fascia over the adductor pollicis; its

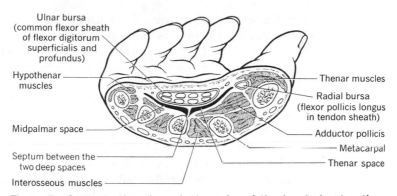

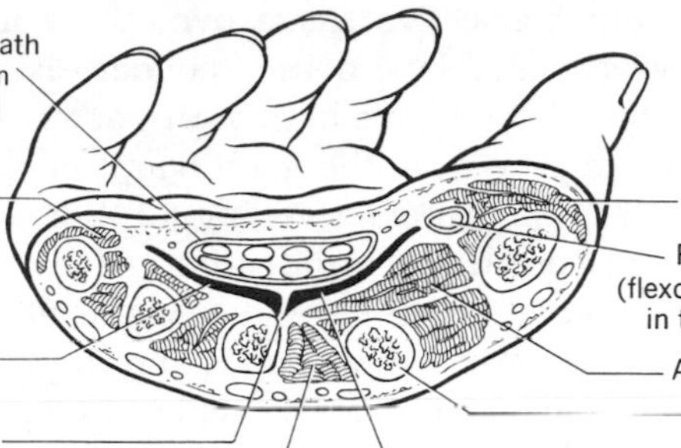

Figure 2—Cross section through the palm of the hand showing the deep spaces and the septum between them. Notice the superficial, deep, medial, and lateral boundaries of the thenar space. Also notice how infection from the radial bursa could spread to the thenar space and vice versa.

lateral boundary is the radial bursa; and medially it is separated from the midpalmar space by a fibrous septum that attaches dorsally to the third metacarpal (Fig. 2). What structure would an infection of the thenar space have to penetrate to spread to the midpalmar space? It would have to rupture through the previously mentioned septum between the two deep spaces.

Lymph drainage of the upper extremity

The edema of the dorsum present early in this case is due to infection of the lymphatic vessels. What course do the lymphatic vessels from the fingers and palm take? Lymph vessels from the palmar and dorsal aspects of the digits drain into a plexus on the dorsum of the hand. From here and from a lymph plexus in the palm of the hand collecting vessels run superficially on the volar aspect of the forearm.

What is the anatomical reason that the edema which accompanies the infection of the lymphatic vessels is more noticeable on the dorsum than in the palm? Remember that the subcutaneous connective tissue over the dorsum is much looser and not confined by a dense aponeurosis as in the palm. What indication do you have in this case of progressive lymph vessel infection? Where are the main lymph nodes draining the hand located? The marked swelling of the axillary lymph nodes indicates spread of the infection via lymphatic vessels to the main collecting station for the lymph of the upper extremity.

Are there any lymph nodes interposed between the hand and the axillary nodes? The cubital (supratrochlear) nodes in the medial bicipital groove three fingerbreadths above the cubital fossa act as an intermediate drainage station for lymph coming from the medial three fingers and the medial side of the hand and forearm. They drain into the axillary nodes. Of the five groups of axillary nodes, that is, the lateral, pectoral, subscapular, central, and apical groups, which one is the primary recipient of lymph from the upper extremity? The lateral group located medial and posterior to the axillary vein receives most of the lymph from the upper limb and drains into the central and apical nodes. A few lymph vessels follow the course of the cephalic vein and drain into deltopectoral nodes in the triangle of the same name and from there into the apical nodes.

37 Carpal Tunnel Syndrome

A 55-year-old seamstress consults her physician, complaining of tingling and burning pain over the volar aspect of thumb, index, middle, and lateral side of ring finger of her right hand. The symptoms began gradually over the last two years and lately have become more intense. They are most marked during the night, keeping her awake. She complains that in getting up in the morning her fingers feel puffy and stiff, but her symptoms gradually subside during the morning. However, if she overworks, particularly if she does heavy ironing, the pain and discomfort increase again. Recently she experiences difficulties in holding on to tableware, resulting in frequent breakage. She also can hardly keep her grasp on the sewing needle. At the same time, she notices that the movements of her right thumb are not as strong as before. This is accompanied by some wasting in the outer half of the ball of this thumb. For the last few weeks, she also complains of occasional burning in the corresponding area of thumb and fingers of her left hand.

EXAMINATION

On inspection of her right hand, flattening of the outer half of the thenar eminence is noticed. On testing, there is loss of power and limitation of range of motion on abduction and opposition of the thumb. Diminished sensibility (hypesthesia and hypalgesia) over the volar aspect of thumb, index, middle, and lateral aspect of the ring finger on the right is demonstrated by impaired appreciation of light touch and pin pricks, and decreased differentiation between sharp and blunt stimuli. Sensation over the lateral aspect of the palm including the thenar eminence is unaffected. Pressure and tapping over the lateral portion of the flexor retinaculum cause tingling and a sensation of "pins and needles" in the involved fingers. On study of the motor functions of the muscles of the right forearm and fingers, no interference with active motion of elbow, wrist, and fingers (except for the described deficiencies in the motion of the thumb) is noted. But, extreme flexion and extension of the wrist reproduces the typical pain in the lateral three and one-half digits of her hand.

DIAGNOSIS

Carpal tunnel syndrome.

THERAPY AND FURTHER COURSE

Since the patient rejects immediate surgery, conservative treatment with immobilization of the wrist during the night by splinting and physical therapy with heat, massage, and mild exercises are tried for several weeks, but have no effect. Anti-inflammatory treatment with hydrocortisone injections also does not lead to any improvement. Thus, surgical treatment consisting of division of the flexor retinaculum is agreed upon. Under local anesthesia, with a tourniquet around the upper arm to obtain a bloodless surgical field, the flexor retinaculum is divided with attention to and avoidance of the superficial palmar vascular arch and the motor or recurrent branch of the median nerve. At operation the synovial sheath of the flexor tendons beneath the flexor retinaculum appears swollen with the median nerve being somewhat flattened and compressed in the narrowest part of the carpal tunnel. This decompression operation results in dramatic disappearance of her pain and other subjective symptoms and gradual cessation of the sensory deficiencies in the next few months. Motor recovery also occurs, although somewhat later.

Since the patient is right-handed and can now use her dominant hand without hindrance, the symptoms on the left side also gradually subside.

DISCUSSION

Sensory deficiencies

This patient offers the subjective symptoms of paresthesias (tingling and numbness) and pain in the lateral three and one-half digits of her right hand, as well as the objective signs of sensory loss, including loss of pain perception on painful stimulation, over approximately the same cutaneous area. How do you explain the apparently contradictory finding of spontaneous pain and interference with pain perception in approximately the same area? The former is an irritative phenomenon due to stimulation of certain sensory nerve fibers while the latter is an indication of destruction and loss of function of certain other sensory fibers. This is a frequent combination in neurological disorders.

Motor deficiencies

There is a loss of motor function of the short abductor and opponens pollicis, combined with wasting at the site of these two muscles in the lateral part of the ball of the right thumb. What is the function of the abductor pollicis brevis and opponens pollicis and how do you test their action? Since it is the function of the abductor pollicis brevis to pull the thumb away from the palm in a plane at right angles to it, you ask the patient to point the thumb toward the ceiling against resistance, seeing to it that the forearm is supine and the dorsum of the hand resting on a table. The opponens pollicis pulls the thumb across the hand in an arch, rotating it at the same time, so that at the end of the motion the palmar surface of thumb and little finger are in opposition to each other. Testing is done accordingly by letting the patient execute this motion against the resistance of your outstretched finger.

Location of the site of the lesion

Where then is the site of the lesion that causes the combined sensory and motor deficiencies? We can exclude systemic diseases of the central nervous system, such as multiple sclerosis, which cause more widespread impairments than are present in our case. We can likewise rule out involvement of a spinal nerve before its division into ventral and dorsal primary rami at the site of the intervertebral foramen, since there is no indication of sensory or motor deficiencies on the dorsal aspect of the trunk supplied by dorsal primary rami. By contrast, it might be tempting in our case, to place the lesion in one or more ventral primary rami in the neck, where they form the roots and trunks of the brachial plexus. Until recently this was assumed to be the site of deficiences of this nature. What roots or trunks of the brachial plexus would have to be involved? A dermatome chart would place the sensory deficiencies in the ventral rami of C6 and C7 which form part of the upper and all of the middle trunk of the brachial plexus. On the other hand, the weight of neurological evidence indicates that the muscles affected in our case, the abductor pollicis brevis and the opponens pollicis, receive their motor supply from the segments C8 and T1, by way of the median nerve. It would have to be a widespread lesion, involving practically all roots of the brachial plexus from C6 to T1, to accommodate all deficiencies in our case. In view of the limited extent of the neurological defect this seems very unlikely. Consequently, we have to assume that the lesion is more peripheral than the brachial plexus.

Is there a peripheral nerve in the upper extremity which supplies the two affected muscles and the skin of the lateral three and one-half digits on their volar aspect? The median nerve innervates the abductor pollicis brevis and opponens pollicis, as well as the involved skin.

Level of median nerve involvement

At what level would the median nerve have to be interrupted to cause the defects present in this case? In other words, where can we pinpoint the lesion that causes the described impairments but leaves the other important motor and sensory functions of the median nerve intact?

Does the median nerve supply any muscles in the arm or forearm? While it does not innervate any muscles in the arm, it supplies the flexors and pronators of the forearm, the flexors of the wrist (with the exception of the flexor carpi ulnaris), and the long flexors of the fingers (with the exception of the medial two bellies of the flexor digitorum profundus). Since the muscles of the forearm supplied by the median nerve display normal function in our patient, the lesion must be located distal to the origin of the branches to these muscles but proximal to the origin of the motor nerve to the opponens pollicis and the abductor pollicis brevis. Where is this branch given off? It is often called the recurrent branch of the median nerve and leaves the lateral side of the nerve as the latter emerges from beneath the flexor retinaculum (Fig. 1). It runs superficial to or through the substance of the flexor pollicis brevis to supply the two muscles of the thumb involved in our case. The same nerve also supplies the superficial portion of the flexor pollicis brevis, but its loss of function cannot be demonstrated by ordinary clinical testing. This also holds true for the lateral two lumbrical muscles which likewise receive their nerve supply from the terminal portion of the median nerve but via the otherwise sensory first two common palmar digital branches. The action of other muscles such as the interossei, which are supplied by the ulnar nerve, obscures the deficiency of the lumbrical muscles. By contrast, clinical experience proves that the abducting action of the abductor pollicis longus, innervated by the radial nerve, is not strong enough to compensate for the paralyzed abductor pollicis brevis.

Can we derive similar localizing indications from the sensory deficiencies in our case history? We notice that sensation over the lateral aspect of the palm and the thenar eminence is unaffected. What cutaneous nerve supplies this area and where is it given off the median nerve? The palmar cutaneous branch arises from the median nerve just proximal to the upper margin of the flexor retinaculum and supplies the uninvolved skin of palm and thenar eminence (Fig. 1). By contrast, the terminal sensory branches of the median nerve supply the skin of the lateral three and one-half digits that display the sensory loss. Therefore, we can pinpoint the lesion in that portion of the median nerve located below the origin of the unaffected palmar cutaneous branch but above its terminal division into the three common palmar digital branches.

One final question in regard to localization of the level of the lesion within the median nerve has to be answered. Why can our deficiency not be caused by a circumscribed injury to the median nerve more proximally in the arm or forearm? One might assume that such a lesion could affect just that component of the nerve that farther distally forms the terminal portion of the nerve involved in our case. This hypothesis presupposes that the fascicles of nerve fibers, which are seen on cross-section of the median and other peripheral nerves, correspond to branches of the main nerve that are given off farther distally and that such fascicles remain intact in their composition within the main nerve trunk throughout its course. This simple "cable" theory has been disproved. It has been shown that within the nerve the identity of a given sensory or motor branch is preserved only for a few centimeters proximal to the origin of the branch from the main stem. Through the intermediation of intraneural plexuses the various fascicles, which make up the main nerve, change their composition continuously by divisions and anastomoses so that the aggregations of nerve fibers composing a given branch are distributed over various fascicles a few centimeters proximal to the point where the branch emerges from the main stem. Thus, it will be impossible to identify the sensory and motor nerve fibers that supply the lateral three and one-half digits and the two muscles of the thumb in a circumscribed cross-sectional area of the median nerve in the arm or proximal forearm. They are dispersed throughout the cross section of the median nerve so that a lesion at any higher level could not imitate a peripheral injury to a branch of this nerve.

Summarizing this discussion on the localization of the defect

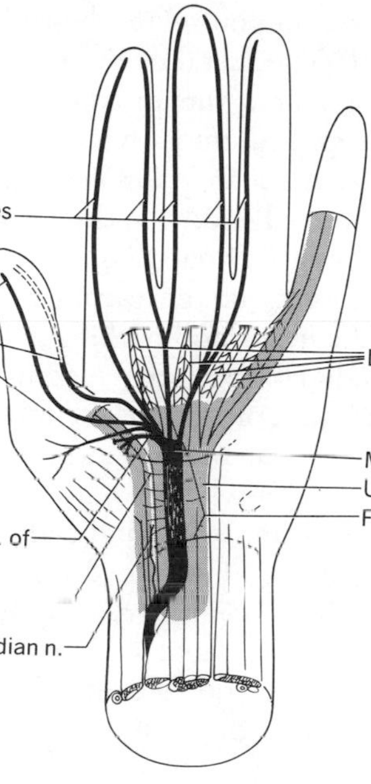

Figure 1—Median nerve in carpal tunnel and its distribution in palm of hand.

within the median nerve, we have to place it in the nerve where it runs through the carpal tunnel. This is a common site for median nerve involvement that has been known to clinicians for only the last 20 years, and is called the "carpal tunnel syndrome." What is the carpal tunnel?

Definition and contents of the carpal tunnel

The carpel tunnel is a a fibro-osseous canal whose trough is formed by the volar concavity of the carpal bones and whose roof consists of the flexor retinaculum, a rigid, inelastic ligament. What are the attachments of the flexor retinaculum? The latter extends from the scaphoid and trapezium on the lateral side to the pisiform and hook of the hamate on the medial side. How would you relate the retinaculum to the skin creases in the hand? The distal of the two creases on the volar aspect of the wrist marks the proximal margin of the flexor retinaculum. The retinaculum is two to three centimeters long, and nearly as wide. A rectangular postage stamp of this size, laid with its narrower edge on the distal crease, would outline the area occupied by the retinaculum.

What are the contents of the carpal tunnel or canal? They are the tendon of the flexor pollicis longus in its synovial sheath (also called the radial bursa), the tendons of the flexor digitorum superficialis and profundus in their common synovial sheath (the so-called ulnar bursa), and the median nerve (Figs. 1 and 2). The latter, with which we are concerned in this case history, lies lateral to the two superficial tendons of the flexor digitorum superficialis against the deep surface of the flexor retinaculum. Does the median nerve supply the muscles listed as contents of the carpal canal with motor fibers within the carpal tunnel? It does not do so, since the motor nerve supply to a muscle has to reach the muscle in its contractile portion, not at its tendon or tendons. The muscle bellies of the indicated muscles are located higher up in the forearm.

Reasons for compression of median nerve

The carpal tunnel, being occupied by the structures listed and being covered by a rigid ligament, appears crowded as it is. Thus, it is not surprising that any space-occupying alteration within the canal, such as a chronic inflammation of the synovial sheath of the common flexor tendons, leads to compression of the median nerve. This would explain the clinical signs and symptoms of irritation and paralysis of the median nerve described in our case. The inflammation of the synovial sac of the common flexor tendon sheath, a so-called tenosynovitis, is probably caused in our patient by occupational strain and overexertion. It is not surprising that the symptoms are aggravated by motions that increase the pressure within the tunnel such as hyperflexion and hyperextension. Hormonal disturbances, such as myxedema and acromegaly, that lead to

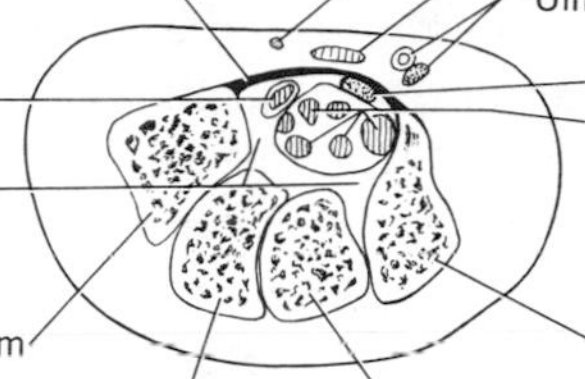

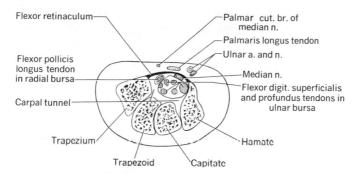

Figure 2—Proximal view of left carpal tunnel showing structures in tunnel and superficial to flexor retinaculum.

waterlogging and deposition of additional connective tissue in the carpal tunnel, also compress the median nerve. Fluid retention, which often accompanies pregnancy, may have the same effect. Increase in clinical symptoms during the night can be explained on the basis of venous stasis during the hours of rest.

Some authors have explained the median nerve deficiency not by direct compression of the nerve itself, but rather by interference with its blood supply due to pressure on the vasa nervorum. Others ascribe the nerve symptoms to increase in endoneural and perineural connective tissue within the nerve, such as might occur in older age groups and also through possible scarring and shrinkage of the endoneural supporting tissue.

Surgically endangered structures superficial to the flexor retinaculum

Identify the structures that run superficial to the flexor retinaculum and that have to be guarded against injury at the time of surgery (Fig. 2). The superficial palmar arterial arch has been mentioned. What vessels form it? Its main component is the superficial branch of the ulnar artery, covered by the palmar carpal ligament. This artery meets the superficial palmar branch of the radial artery or more rarely the radial branch to the index finger or the princeps pollicis branch. The palmar cutaneous branches of the median and ulnar nerves accompany the tendon of the palmaris longus as it passes superficial to the flexor retinaculum. The danger to the recurrent motor branch of the median, which is given off distal to the flexor retinaculum, has been mentioned previously.

Other nerve entrapments

In recent years attention has been drawn to other areas where due to their anatomical configuration nerve entrapments take place. The cause is generally compression of a nerve where it runs through an inelastic fibrous ring or a rigid fibro-osseous tunnel. The compression may be due to a local condition such as callus formation after fracture or rheumatoid arthritis, bursitis, or synovitis with swelling. Systemic diseases such as hypothyroidism, acromegaly, or collagen disorders may also cause nerve compression by waterlogging and deposition of connective tissue in an already crowded space. In addition to the carpal tunnel such a condition occurs where the median nerve runs between the two heads of the pronator teres and dips under a fibrous band that connects the two heads of the flexor digitorum superficialis. The ulnar nerve may be entrapped at the wrist in a trough where it passes between the pisiform and hook of hamate. The same nerve may also be compressed in the ulnar groove behind the medial epicondyle. Other entrapment neuropathies, as these conditions are called, occur in the posterior interosseous nerve of the radial as it passes through the supinator muscle, in the suprascapular nerve within the suprascapular foramen, in the common and superficial peroneal nerves, and in the tibial nerve beneath the flexor retinaculum in the so-called tarsal tunnel.

Lower Extremity

38 Intragluteal Injection

A 39-year-old carpenter suffered a respiratory infection with high fever and cough and was given several penicillin injections into his buttocks by a nurse in a physician's office. Immediately after the last injection into his right buttock he complained of numbness, tingling, and burning in his right leg down to his toes and developed a foot drop the next day, when he was hospitalized.

EXAMINATION

On examination at the hospital it is found that his respiratory infection has almost cleared up. His fever and cough have subsided and the physical findings in his lungs are minimal.

Inspection of the right gluteal region shows several injection marks approximately over the course of the right sciatic nerve slightly above the gluteal fold.

The sensory loss involves the outer side of the right calf and the dorsum of the right foot. On the motor side there is inability to dorsiflex the ankle and to evert the foot, with noticeable foot drop. There also is difficulty in extending the toes. On walking the patient drags the front part and outer margin of his foot.

DIAGNOSIS

Respiratory infection with neural complications arising from intramuscular injections.

THERAPY AND FURTHER COURSE

The patient is given deep heat followed by electrical stimulation of the involved muscles and reeducation exercises. After four months he has essentially regained the motor functions of his right leg but still shows some sensory deficiencies.

DISCUSSION

What is the surface marking of the sciatic nerve at the level of the gluteal fold? It is approximately midway between greater trochanter and ischial tuberosity, but somewhat closer to the latter. Of the two components of the sciatic nerve, the tibial and the common peroneal, which part seems exclusively involved in this case? The greater susceptibility of the common peroneal nerve in injuries of the sciatic nerve is a characteristic feature which has often been observed. It is explained by the fact that the common peroneal component is placed more superficially, indicating a slight rotation of the sciatic nerve. Histological evidence reveals that the bundles of nerve fibers in the common peroneal nerve are larger in size but fewer in number and are enclosed in a smaller amount of protective connective tissue than those in the tibial nerve. This might also be a reason for the greater vulnerability of the common peroneal nerve. In addition, the more lateral location of this nerve makes it more liable to injuries by intramuscular injection, which, according to standard rules, is directed into the upper lateral quadrant of the gluteal region.

How does the sciatic nerve enter the gluteal region? What is its usual relation to the piriformis muscle? It usually enters the gluteal region distal to this muscle ("infrapiriform"). In 15 per cent of cases, however, the common peroneal division of the sciatic nerve passes above or through the piriformis muscle instead of below it increasing the danger to this division in cases where this variation is present.

Neural deficiencies

What sensory branch of the common peroneal nerve is responsible for the loss of sensation over the lateral side of the calf? The lateral sural cutaneous nerve, a branch of the common peroneal, supplies this area with sensory fibers. How do you account for the loss of sensation on the dorsum of the foot? Cutaneous branches of the superficial peroneal nerve (medial and intermediate dorsal) transmit sensation from the dorsum of the foot. What named nerve is responsible for dorsiflexion of the foot and extension of the toes? The deep peroneal nerve innervates the dorsiflexors of the foot and extensors of the toes. Is this the same nerve that mediates sensation from the dorsal aspect of the foot? It is not. What nerve effectuates eversion of the foot? The peroneus longus and brevis muscles are the main evertors of the foot and are supplied by the superficial peroneal nerve. Would loss of function of only one of the two terminal branches of the common peroneal nerve explain all the neurological deficiencies? The sensory and motor deficiencies in this case can be explained only on the basis of involvement of the main stem, that is, the common peroneal nerve.

Applied anatomy of intragluteal injections

The gluteal region is a common site for intramuscular application of drugs. Intramuscular rather than intravenous injections are given when prolonged action is preferred to immediate effect. They are more easily administered and are often better tolerated. In addition, oily preparations cannot be injected directly into the bloodstream but can be given intramuscularly. Irritant drugs are excluded from the otherwise simpler subcutaneous application, where they may cause sloughing or abscess formation. The rich blood supply of the heavy gluteal musculature makes this area a favorable site of parenteral (non-gastrointestinal) administration of drugs. Name the main arteries and veins supplying this region. The superior and inferior gluteal vessels are the essential vessels in this area.

How would you avoid the inadvertent application of drugs into the subcutaneous tissue or the even more dangerous penetration of the medium into the gluteal vessels? Keep in mind that the subcutaneous adipose layer over the gluteal area

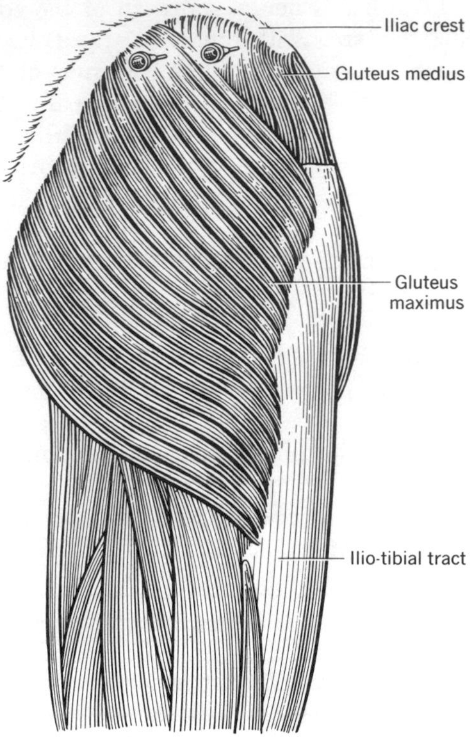

Figure 1—Superficial aspect of musculature of gluteal region. Two needles for intramuscular injection are in place in upper outer quadrant in gluteus maximus and medius.

varies greatly in thickness and may reach a depth of two and one-half inches, particularly in women. The injection needle will, of course, have to penetrate beyond this layer if painful indurations and abscesses are to be avoided. Intravenous application into one of the gluteal veins should be guarded against by slightly withdrawing the plunger of the syringe and inspecting the syringe for blood. What would the result be if an oily suspension were injected into one of the thin-walled gluteal veins? Identify all named components of the cardiovascular system such an embolus (plug) would traverse until it reaches the lung where it might cause dangerous or even fatal complications.

Such an oil embolus would travel via the gluteal veins into the internal and common iliac veins, the inferior vena cava, the right atrium and ventricle, and the pulmonary artery to be arrested in the pulmonary circulation.

Even more dangerous is the inadvertent injection into the gluteal arteries. Such an accident may lead to drug emboli in the cutaneous branches leading to painful swelling of the skin and subcutaneous tissue and necrosis (tissue death). If the drug is injected into a gluteal artery under high pressure, the embolus may be directed against the bloodstream into the internal iliac artery and its visceral branches with even more dangerous and occasional fatal results such as gangrene of bladder, vagina, penis, or rectum.

If, as stipulated, the injection is made into the upper outer quadrant of the gluteal region, it is given either into the gluteus maximus or the gluteus medius, depending on whether the solution is injected into the lower inner or the upper outer portion of this quadrant (Fig. 1). Which direction of the needle should be avoided in order to prevent injury to the sciatic nerve? It is clear that injection downward and medially would be most apt to reach the sciatic nerve. Since a relaxed muscle admits the injected fluid without back pressure, in what position of the lower extremity should the gluteus maximus, a powerful lateral rotator of the hip, be injected? This is the reason why many physicians recommend the "toed-in" position or medial rotation of the extremity.

Injury to superior and inferior gluteal nerves

Two other motor nerves, the superior and inferior gluteal nerves, are occasionally damaged by intragluteal injection. Where in relation to the piriformis muscle does the superior gluteal nerve leave the greater sciatic foramen? Can you explain why it is only rarely injured although it ramifies in the upper outer quadrant? Does it run between gluteus maximus

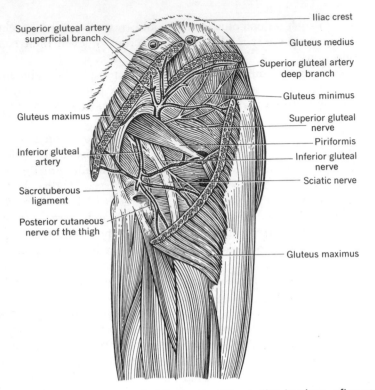

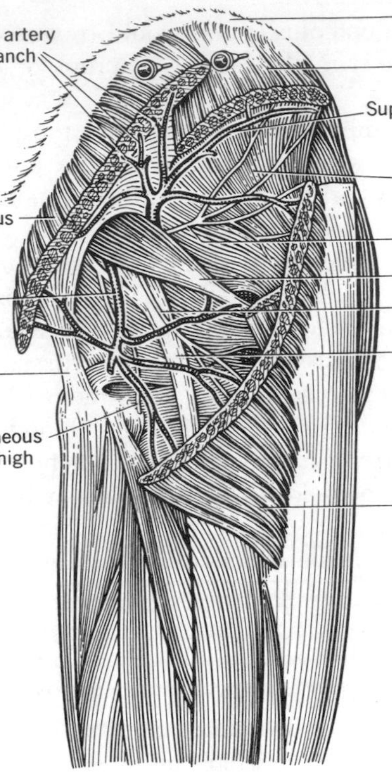

Figure 2—Anatomy of gluteal area with needles in place, after partial section of gluteus maximus and medius. Shown are sciatic nerve and superior and inferior gluteal arteries and nerves. Notice that both gluteal arteries, but only the inferior gluteal nerve, supply the gluteus maximus. The superior gluteal nerve lies on the deep aspect of the gluteus medius, between it and the minimus and supplies both muscles.

and medius or deep to the medius? It leaves the pelvis above the piriformis ("suprapiriform") and runs between gluteus medius and minimus, both of which it supplies (Fig. 2). The deep location and the early branching of this nerve close to its exit from the pelvis seem to explain the rarity of complications originating from injections. Does the same deep location also characterize all branches of the superior gluteal vessels?

The superior gluteal vessels have superficial branches which run between the gluteus maximus and medius.

Which is the nerve of supply to the gluteus maximus? This nerve, the inferior gluteal, may likewise be damaged in improperly located injections. While the inferior gluteal nerve is the only source of supply for this most powerful muscle in the human body, is this also true for the inferior gluteal vessels? The superficial branches of the superior gluteal artery and vein, in addition to the inferior gluteal vessels, participate in the supply of the gluteus maximus muscle and are endangered in subgluteal injections (Fig. 2).

Other locations of intramuscular injections

Scrupulous adherence to all rules governing intramuscular injections has to be observed to avoid serious and often lasting complications. Other muscle sites that have been recommended are the quadriceps femoris, vastus lateralis, deltoid (here serious neurological mishaps have likewise been reported), and recently the more anterior aspects of the gluteus medius and minimus, caudal and posterior to the anterior superior spine of the ilium.

39 Intracapsular Hip Fracture

A 72-year-old widow, who lives with her oldest son, was found on the floor of her bedroom, unable to rise. She told her son that she had slipped on a scatter rug and had fallen to the floor. She complained of severe pain in her right hip and was unable to stand up. Since no physician was immediately available, an ambulance was called, and she was taken to the hospital on a stretcher. On arrival she was given a small dose of morphine and was made more comfortable by immobilization of her limb with pillows and sandbags, and by bandages that held her two legs together.

EXAMINATION

The patient is a frail, elderly woman in rather poor nutritional state. Her muscles are poorly developed. Mentally she is somewhat confused, which could be ascribed to the shock and the narcotic. Physical examination reveals that her right leg is externally rotated and that she is unable to lift her right heel from the stretcher. The right leg seems shortened. This is confirmed by measuring the distance between the anterior superior iliac spine and the distal tip of the medial malleolus of the tibia with a tape measure and by comparing the results with those obtained in the left leg, which is rotated into the same position as the right. There is shortening of her right leg by one and one-half inches. The greater trochanter on the right side appears higher and more prominent than the left.

On palpation there is tenderness in the femoral triangle in front of the hip joint.

DIAGNOSIS

A presumptive diagnosis of fracture through the femoral neck is made and the patient's hip is roentgenographed in two directions. This procedure confirms the diagnosis and demonstrates the fracture just below the head of the femur (subcapital). The neck of the femur points forward and the angle between head and neck of the femur is decreased (varus deformity). Neck and shaft are externally rotated and the fragments overlap with the neck and shaft having moved cranially against the head (Fig. 1). The pelvic skeleton and femur show marked demineralization (osteoporosis).

THERAPY AND FURTHER COURSE

In our aged patient who is in poor nutritional state, there is great danger of bed sores, urinary infection, pneumonia, and pulmonary embolism with possible fatal outcome, if the malposition of the fracture is corrected by closed reduction and the patient is confined to her bed with the limb immobilized until the fracture had a chance to heal. The head of the femur, when separated from its neck, has a poor blood supply left in subcapital location of the fracture. Consequently, nonunion of the fragments and late necrosis are likely to occur. These complications frequently lead to secondary degenerative osteoarthritis resulting in a painful and disabled hip.

Thus, in view of the poor prognosis of conservative treatment in our patient, immediate surgery with removal of the femoral head and replacement with a vitallium prosthesis is decided upon. Vitallium is an extremely hard alloy which is supposed to be electrically neutral and therefore well tolerated by bone and surrounding tissues. The prosthesis chosen in this case not only replaces the head, but also has a long stem that is inserted into the bone-marrow cavity almost halfway down the femoral shaft to anchor the head. The stem of the prosthesis is fenestrated (has windows) and bits of cancellous bone, removed from the upper end of the femur, are placed in these windows as bone grafts. It is expected that these bone chips will become converted into dense, new osseous tissue, locking the prosthesis in place and lending strength and stability to the femoral shaft for its weight-bearing function.

Under spinal anesthesia the hip is approached by a skin and fascial incision through the lower part of the buttocks. The gluteus maximus is split in the direction of its fibers by blunt dissection. Only its lower fibers are divided vertical to their direction. The upper and lower portions of this muscle are separated and retracted, thus exposing the sciatic nerve and the lateral rotators of the hip. The latter are divided close to their insertion into the greater trochanter. After removal of the overlying fat the capsule is incised and partly reflected. The head of the femur is dislodged out of the acetabulum and removed. The ligamentum teres is ligated and excised. The neck of the femur is sawed across and the stem of a well-fitting vitallium prosthesis is inserted into the marrow cavity. Care is taken to preserve the normal forward angle of neck and head. A tight fit of the prosthesis is obtained after moving the artificial head into place.

The operation lasts about thirty-five minutes and the patient is able to sit up in bed and eat on the afternoon of the day of operation. After four days the patient is up and around on crutches and leaves the hospital after ten days. She is cautioned to use crutches and only partial weight bearing is permitted for about six months. She is re-examined and roentgenographed at frequent intervals and is told to use a cane for the remainder of her life. She is also warned not to expose her leg to too much strain and to avoid heavy weight gain.

On re-examination after a year, the patient reports that she can do her own housework and can walk with no limp or pain. She has practically normal function of her hip.

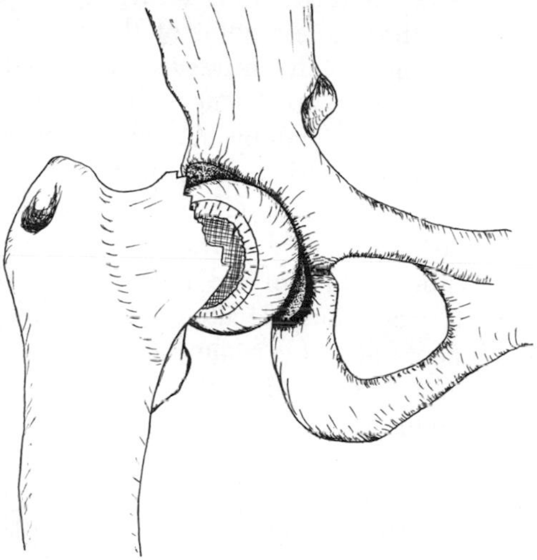

Figure 1—Intracapsular subcapital fracture through the neck of the femur. The neck of the femur points forward and neck and shaft are externally rotated. Notice the decrease in the angle between head and neck (varus deformity).

DISCUSSION

The anatomy of intra- and extracapsular fractures of the neck of the femur

We are dealing here with a very common clinical condition of the elderly, particularly the female where a neck fracture is ten times more common than in the male. In many cases the fracture is the direct cause of death, as discussed in the case history. Modern advances in the handling of these fractures include insertion of a prosthesis, as in our case, or the nailing of the fragments, depending on the judgment and preference of the surgeon. These procedures have resulted in avoidance of general complications by allowing early ambulation and quite frequently have given good functional results.

As described previously in the case history, the rotational strain in slipping had caused a fracture with complete separation of the fragments. The fracture line is located just below the head of the femur at the highest point of the neck (subcapital) and is therefore completely intracapsular. What are the attachments of the capsule? Are all neck fractures intracapsular? The fibrous capsule, lined by synovial membrane, arises from the margins of the acetabulum of the hip bone and extends sleevelike downward and laterally around the neck of the femur to attach near the intertrochanteric line anteriorly and close to the middle of the neck posteriorly, a fingerbreadth above the posteriorly located intertrochanteric crest. From the attachments of the capsule the synovial membrane is reflected on to the neck and up to the margin of the articular cartilage which, as in all other joints, is not covered by synovia.

From this description we realize that the lateral and distalmost portions of the posterior aspect of the neck are outside the capsule, so that neck fractures, in contrast to the injury in our case, may be partly intra-, partly extracapsular. Intertrochanteric fractures are always extracapsular.

The anatomy of displacement of the fragments

What is the typical position of the fractured extremity and how do you explain this position? Typically the leg is externally rotated due to the pull of the lateral rotators and the weight of the leg and foot itself. Which are the lateral rotators? They are the short muscles within the gluteal region, i.e. the piriformis, the obturator internus and externus, the gemelli and the quadratus femoris which are aided by the gluteus maximus. The external rotators are much more powerful than the internal which explains the position of the leg.

How do you explain the shortening of the extremity in our case? The force of the injury itself may drive the distal fragment cranially, but in general it is the muscle pull that leads to this result. Identify the muscles whose pull causes shortening of the leg. The powerful gluteal muscles, the hamstrings, the adductors, the ileopsoas, and some of the flexors of the thigh, all these arise from the pelvis or lumbar spinal column above the fracture line and insert into the distal fragment. Their pull results in upward displacement of the lower fragment and shortening of the leg.

Angles of inclination and declination

The muscle pull also leads to a change in the angle of femoral head and neck with the shaft. Normally this angle is about 130°, being larger in the child. This is the so-called angle of inclination. As so often in hip fractures, the roentgenogram in our case reveals that the angle is reduced resulting in what is called a coxa vara (Fig. 1). By contrast, an occasional fracture through the neck may take place in abduction of the thigh at the time of injury. If this happens, the neck will be driven in the abducted position into the head where it remains firmly impacted. This increases the angle of inclination and results in the so-called valgus position. Such a fracture has a better prognosis. There is no shortening of the leg and very little pain.

Also of importance is the anteriorly open angle between neck and shaft of the femur, the so-called angle of declination. In contrast to the shoulder where the head of the humerus faces posteriorly, the head and neck of the femur are directed anteriorly. This angle between the planes laid through neck and shaft is normally about 12°, and care has to be taken to preserve it in setting the neck fracture or inserting the prosthesis. Any marked alteration in the angles of inclination and declination may seriously interfere with mobility of the hip joint and disable the patient.

Other important anatomical angles

Although anatomical textbooks generally do not stress the subject, the physician who sets fractures has to be aware of these angles in many bones to avoid interference with proper joint function. Only a few important examples will be given here. While the carrying angle of the elbow is well known and covered in the textbook literature, there is a less well-known but equally important anteriorly open angle of 30 to 60° between the long axis of the shaft of the humerus and its distal articular end. Disregard of this angle in reduction of condylar and supracondylar fractures and epiphyseal separations will lead to loss of flexion and severe disability of the elbow joint. If in the setting of Colles' fracture, no attention is paid to the normal palmar tilt of the distal end of the radius which amounts to an angle of 10 to 15° between the articular surface of this bone and its long axis, there is considerable loss of function in the wrist joint. Finally, attention should be called to the normal angle between the anterior-superior and posterior-superior surfaces of the calcaneus. This posteriorly open calcaneal angle is normally 25 to 40°. In common crash fractures of this largest and most important bone of the foot, this angle is decreased or reversed through flattening of the bone. If this deformity is disregarded in the treatment of calcaneal fracture, severe and permanent disability results.

Blood supply of the shaft, neck, and head of the femur

A problem that has direct bearing on the course and handling of our fracture is the blood supply to the proximal portion of the femur. Long bones such as the femur are well supplied with blood vessels. These are derived from the following three sources: (1) the nutrient artery, which enters the bone through the nutrient foramen. The artery takes an oblique course through the cortex of the bone until it reaches the marrow cavity where it divides into ascending and descending branches. The nutrient artery is largely concerned with supply of the bone marrow and the inner two-thirds of the cortex. In the femur, there are two nutrient foramina and the nutrient arteries passing into them are derived from the perforating branches of the deep femoral artery. (2) Periosteal vessels, which in the periosteum form a communicating network that surrounds the bone. The number of periosteal vessels increases from the middle of the diaphysis toward the metaphyses which are richly supplied with blood vessels. Fine branches of the periosteal network enter the outer third of the cortical bone and anastomose with vessels derived from the nutrient artery in the inner portion of the cortex. The two systems of the nutritional and periosteal blood vessels may partially substitute for each other if the circulation in one or the other system is interrupted. (3) The most important system for the blood supply of the femoral head and neck is the epiphyseal-metaphyseal vascular network. Although minor anastomoses with nutritional and periosteal vessels of the shaft seem to have been demonstrated, the nutrient artery contributes very little or nothing to the blood supply of the head, neck, and trochanters of the femur. The main artery of supply to the head is the medial femoral circumflex, which is commonly listed as a branch of the deep femoral, although variations in its origin occur. By injection studies it was found that the posterosuperior branches of the medial femoral circumflex artery represent the most important blood supply to the head. These vessels, arising from a posterior branch of the medial femoral circumflex, that passes behind the femoral neck, pierce the fibrous capsule of the hip joint and run upward and medially along the posterior and superior aspects of the neck. There they course beneath the synovia surrounding the neck to enter the head through bony foramina close to the site of the former epiphysis. These vessels have also been called retinacular vessels since they lie within easily movable folds or retinacula of the synovial membrane that is reflected from the attachment of the fibrous capsule on to the neck. Other branches enter the head medio-inferiorly to the old epiphyseal line to distribute themselves in the inferiomedial portion of the head. The posterosuperior vessels supply two-thirds to four fifths of the head (Fig. 2). Caudally directed branches of the medial femoral circumflex artery supply the former metaphyseal area distal to the obliterated epiphysis. The epiphyseal and metaphyseal branches of the medial femoral circumflex artery freely anastomose. The extracapsular portion of the neck and the trochanteric area also receive branches from the lateral femoral circumflex and the superior gluteal arteries. The first perforating artery, a branch of the deep femoral artery, and the inferior gluteal artery may also contribute to the blood supply of the

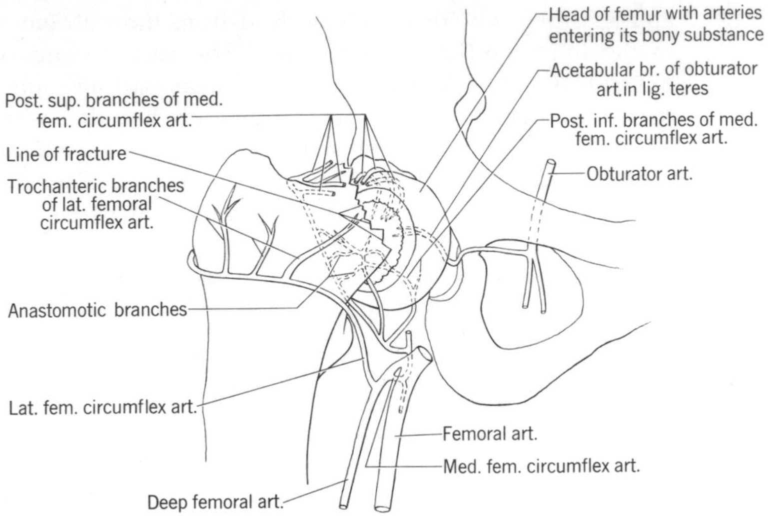

Figure 2—Blood supply of head and neck of femur. Notice that the main artery of supply to the head is the medial femoral circumflex through its posterior-superior and posterior-inferior branches. Also notice the anastomoses between these two systems. Observe that the lateral femoral circumflex artery contributes to the blood supply of the neck. Finally, identify the acetabular branch of the obturator artery which may or may not anastomose with the branches of the medial femoral circumflex artery. Notice also that most of the important arteries to the head have been torn by the fracture, thus compromising the blood supply to the head.

bone. Of great interest is the acetabular branch of the obturator artery that enters the head through the ligamentum teres, which attaches to the fovea of the head. This branch is often called the "foveolar artery." Its extent and patency are variable and its contribution to the blood supply of the head is generally not very significant. The artery may or may not anastomose with the important medially ascending branches of the medial femoral circumflex artery.

Necrosis of the femoral head in subcapital fractures

From the foregoing it is clear that a subcapital fracture, such as is present in our case, leads to tearing of the important retinacular blood vessels beneath the synovia and therefore to interruption of the main blood supply to the head. The nearer the fracture lies to the head the more this is true. On the other hand, trochanteric fractures outside the capsule have a much better chance to allow for sufficient nourishment of the bone. The tenuous blood supply through the vessel in the ligamentum teres generally is insufficient and thus necrosis (tissue death) is more likely to occur the closer the fracture is to the head.

This type of necrosis is due to isolation of the head from its blood supply and is aseptic in contrast to septic necrosis due to bacterial infection.

An interesting radiographic feature of aseptic necrosis of the head is a relative increase in the opacity of the avascular area. This becomes noticeable several weeks or months after the fracture has been sustained. The surrounding area of the neck and shaft becomes increasingly translucent due to bone resorption from disuse and inflammation while the dead head itself, cut off its blood supply, preserves its normal bone density.

Attempts are frequently made to immobilize the fragments by a plaster cast or by nailing, in the hope that the fragments will unite and vessels grow across the fracture line. However, this hope often fails, particularly in subcapital fractures in old patients and the previously described necrosis of the head results. In order to avoid this complication, the head was excised in our case at the time the fracture occurred and was replaced by a prosthesis. Other areas where fractures frequently lead to devascularization and necrosis of one fragment are the scaphoid of the hand and the talus.

Osteoporosis and its underlying anatomy

The roentgenogram of the pelvis of our patient called attention to marked osteoporosis which is so common in the elderly, particularly in the female. What is the cause of this deficiency in the bony framework which in the femoral head and neck leads to noticeable rarefication of the spongy bone and thinning of the cortex and which so often results in fractures from trivial injuries? The true cause of this type of osteoporosis is not clearly understood but it is characterized by a deficiency of the bony matrix. The matrix that is laid down is calcified normally but not enough bony matrix is formed. While we cannot pinpoint the cause of this metabolic change, it seems to be due to an imbalance between gonadal and adrenal cortical hormones.

The surgical anatomy of the operation

The operation done in our patient and briefly described in our history follows the technique suggested by A. T. Moore.[1] What is the direction of the fibers of the gluteus maximus which are split by blunt dissection? The fibers run from medial and cranial to lateral and caudal and only the lowest fibers of the gluteus maximus are cut vertical to this direction to afford access to the hip joint. Does the gluteus maximus insert into the greater trochanter? It passes over the lateral surface of this process, a bursa intervening, and inserts into the iliotibial tract and the gluteal tuberosity, which is an upward extension of the lateral lip of the linea aspera. What is the craniocaudal sequence of the lateral rotator muscles of the hip joint that are in the operative field? They are the piriformis, the superior gemellus, the tendon of the obturator internus, the inferior gemellus, and the quadratus femoris. These are divided in our surgical procedure with the exception of the highest and lowest muscle, the piriformis and quadratus femoris, which are cut only if it is necessary to obtain a wide approach to the joint. The author claims as an advantage of his method that the abductors of the hip joint, that are so important in walking, are not divided and their function is preserved. What are these abductors? They are the gluteus medius and minimus. Another advantage of this approach is the chance to cut the sensory nerves passing from the sciatic nerve and nerve to the quadratus femoris to the hip joint, thus relieving some postoperative pain.

The sensory nerve supply of the hip joint and Hilton's law

A short comment on the sensory nerve supply of the hip joint is indicated since it is responsible for the pain suffered by patients with hip fractures and explains the muscle spasms. An old law formulated by John Hilton [2] is quite applicable to the hip joint, i.e. that a joint receives its proprioceptive and pain fibers from the same nerves which supply the muscles moving the joint and distribute to the skin over these muscles and their insertions. This law also explains the reflex spasm of the overlying muscles in disease of the joint and the referral of joint pain to the adjacent skin. In the hip joint the sensory nerve supply is derived from the femoral, obturator, and sciatic nerves in addition to fibers incorporated in muscular branches to the quadratus femoris.

REFERENCES

1. A. T. Moore, The Self-Locking Metal Hip Prosthesis. J. Bone and Joint Surg. 39A: 811-827, 1957.

2. John Hilton, Rest and Pain, edited by E. W. Walls, E. E. Phillip, and H. J. B. Atkins, Philadelphia: J. B. Lippincott, 1950.

40 "Unhappy Triad" of Knee Joint

A 20-year-old college student, while playing college football, received a twisting injury to his right knee when he was tackled from the side. He experienced immediate excruciating pain in his right knee and had the feeling that something had torn on the inner side of his knee joint. He had to leave the game and one of the trainers strapped the knee with adhesive tape.

EXAMINATION

He is seen the next day by an orthopedist. His knee is markedly swollen, particularly in the suprapatellar region, and held in slight flexion. There is tenderness on pressure along the extent of the tibial collateral ligament. The pain is particularly marked at the tibial attachment of the ligament. Abduction of the leg on the femur aggravates the pain. Roentgenograms under sodium pentothal anesthesia, with the tibia in forceful abduction, show distinct widening of the medial portion of the knee joint space (Fig. 1). When the knee is flexed to a right angle and an attempt made to pull the tibia forward, there is noticeably increased anterior mobility. There is marked restriction of extension of the knee joint.

DIAGNOSIS

A tentative diagnosis is made of an effusion (fluid collection) in the knee joint, rupture of the tibial collateral ligament, with

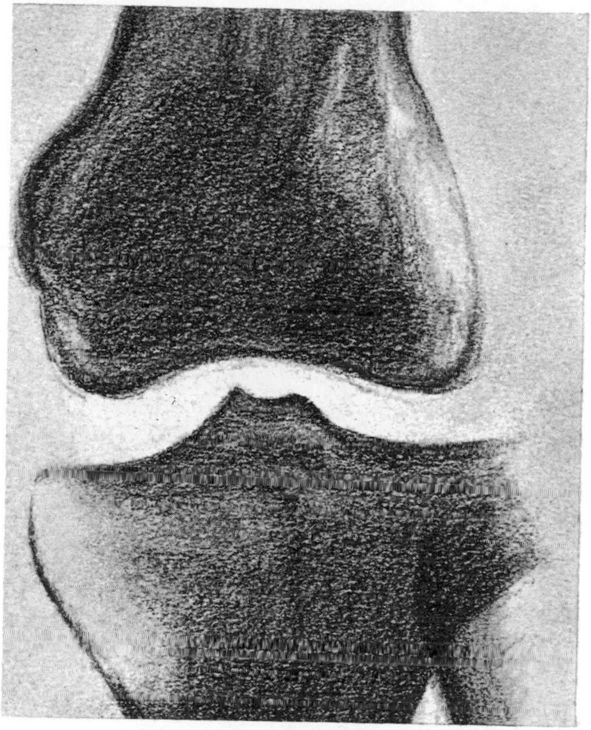

Figure 1 represents anteroposterior roentgenogram taken under anesthesia in forced abduction. Film shows over-all widening of the "joint space" which is caused by the effusion. Greater width of the space on the medial side of the joint is brought about by abduction after tearing of the medial collateral and anterior cruciate ligaments. Keep in mind that the major portion of the roentgenologic joint space is due to invisibility of the articular cartilage on the roentgenogram. Medial and lateral sides of the joint are identified by the presence of the fibula on the lateral side.

probable tear of the anterior cruciate ligament and injury to the medial meniscus.

THERAPY

Surgical exploration under general anesthesia shows that the superficial and deep layers of the tibial collateral ligament

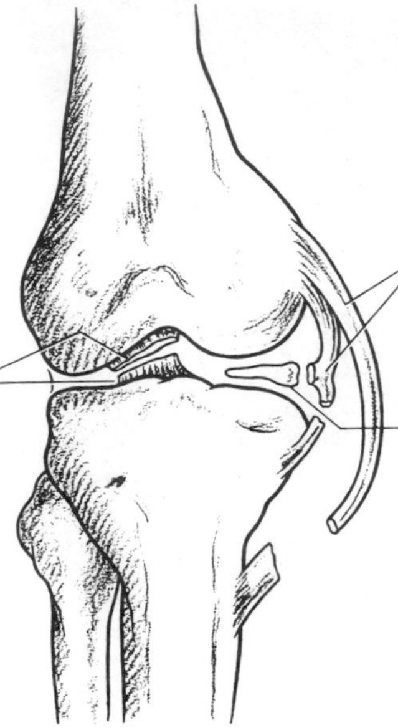

Figure 2 (adapted from O'Donoghue) shows: (1) rupture of the superficial and deep layers of tibial collateral ligament, (2) tear of anterior cruciate ligament, (3) injury to medial meniscus.

have been avulsed from the tibia. The medial meniscus is torn loose from its attachment to the deep layer of the tibial collateral ligament and is lying on the intercondylar surface of the tibia. The anterior cruciate ligament is torn from its posterior attachment to the lateral condyle of the femur (Fig. 2).

The medial meniscus is removed. Both layers of the tibial collateral ligament are anchored by sutures through drill holes in the tibia, and the anterior cruciate ligament is sutured to the site of its original attachment to the femur by anchoring it through drill holes in the bone.

FURTHER COURSE

The knee is fixed in moderate extension by plaster splints extending from the toes to almost the hip and kept immobilized for four weeks. Cotton dressings and splints are applied for another two weeks, during which period the patient is allowed to bear weight on the leg. Thereafter, an elastic bandage for the knee joint is prescribed. Throughout the period, physical therapy is given and graded exercises applied to maintain muscle tone. Later, more vigorous exercises are designed to restore the function of the knee joint.

After a year the patient has a stable knee with no restriction of motion and has resumed his athletic activities.

DISCUSSION

We are dealing here with a not infrequent, nonskeletal injury that has been designated as the "unhappy triad" (O'Donoghue).* What are the three important structures involved? The injury includes. (1) rupture of the tibial collateral ligament; (2) rupture of the anterior cruciate ligament; and (3) damage to the medial meniscus. The effusion present in this case reflects damage to the joint and generally accompanies all types of intra-articular knee joint injuries.

What exaggerated motion caused these injuries in our case? Abduction and lateral rotation of the tibia on the femur through tackling of the running player was responsible.

Movements of the knee joint

Is the knee joint a pure hinge joint allowing only flexion and extension or is some medial and lateral rotation of the leg possible? In what position of the knee would this latter movement be facilitated? In maximal extension the greatest surface areas of femur and tibia are in contact, locking the joint in its most stable position. With increasing flexion the articular surfaces of the two bones lose part of their contact, allowing some rotation but depriving the joint of some of its stability. Was the leg at the time of the injury in its most stable position?

* Don H. O'Donoghue: "Surgical Treatment of Fresh Injuries to the Major Ligaments of the Knee." J. Bone Joint Surg., 32-A:721-738, 1950.

In running, semiflexion takes place, making the knee more liable to ligamentous injury.

Are the articular portions of the femur and tibia sufficiently adapted to each other to make this a stable joint? If the answer is negative, would other elements contribute to the stability of the joint? The joint is surrounded by muscles and tendons and invested by numerous ligaments, which act as the stabilizing element. In addition, the menisci deepen the joint surface of the tibia and accommodate the joint to variations in contact between femur and tibia.

Name the major ligaments which guide the joint through its normal range of motion and, if intact, prevent excessive mobility. They are: the tibial and fibular collateral ligaments, the anterior and posterior cruciate ligaments, the patellar ligament, and the oblique popliteal ligament which reinforces the capsule posteriorly. In this case we are concerned with injuries to two of these ligaments. Identify them.

Tibial collateral ligament

First and foremost, the tibial collateral ligament is involved. What abnormal and excessive motion avulsed the ligament from its attachment to the tibia? Abduction and lateral rotation of the leg, with the knee in partially flexed position, brought about this injury. This motion put more stress on the superficial and deep layers of the ligament than it was able to withstand and it tore off its anchorage to the tibia. What are the attachments of this ligament? Its superficial fibers insert proximally into the medial epicondyle of the femur and distally into the tibial condyle, approximately two inches below its rim. The deep fibers of the ligament are shorter and thicker and connect the inner margins of the medial femoral and tibial condyles. It is to this layer that the medial meniscus is attached. Name the three tendons that cross this ligament. They are the sartorius, gracilis, and semitendinosus, on their way to their common insertion on the proximal portion of the tibia, in front of the attachment of the superficial part of the tibial collateral ligament.

Was the elicited tenderness on pressure in keeping with the

site of the injury? The pain corresponded to the course of the ligament and the area of maximal tenderness to the location of the tear. Did the medial widening of the joint space on the roentgenogram, taken in forceful abduction, confirm the diagnosis of a torn medial collateral ligament (Fig. 1)? It demonstrated the abnormal mobility of the leg in the knee joint and made rupture of the tibial collateral and possibly the anterior cruciate ligaments likely.

Anterior cruciate ligament

The second ligament injured was the anterior cruciate ligament which was torn off its proximal attachment. What are its normal attachments and its function? What is the relation of the cruciate ligaments to the fibrous capsule and synovial membrane? The cruciate ligaments lie inside the capsule but outside the synovial cavity of the joint, the synovial membrane being reflected around them anteriorly and on their sides.

The anterior cruciate ligament is attached cranially to the medial surface of the lateral condyle of the femur. It is directed downward in a medial and anterior direction and inserts on the anterior intercondylar area of the tibia. (If in crossing your legs you swing your right leg over the left, the direction of your right leg parallels that of the right anterior cruciate ligament, from cranial, lateral, and posterior to caudal, medial, and anterior). Review from your text the attachments of the posterior cruciate ligament, which runs posterior to the anterior in the opposite direction. While both cruciate ligaments exert a stabilizing effect on all motions of the knee joint, the anterior limits excessive anterior mobility of the tibia on the femur in extension. How do you explain the avulsion of this ligament in the type of injury encountered in this case? With the foot fixed and the knee semiflexed, a strong force was applied which abducted and laterally rotated the tibia on the femur. As a consequence of this, the anterior cruciate ligament became forcefully stretched over the inner aspect of the medially displaced lateral condyle of the femur and its attachment to the femur was torn.

What clinical sign in the examination of this patient made

tearing of the anterior cruciate ligament quite likely? The increased anterior mobility of the knee in flexion, that was found in our case, is suspicious of rupture of this ligament.

Medial meniscus

The final injury was tearing of the medial meniscus from its attachment to the tibial collateral ligament. What are the shape and the attachments of the medial meniscus? Both menisci are wedge-shaped, being thicker at their peripheral margins. However, in contrast to its lateral counterpart, the medial meniscus forms a small segment of a large circle, that is, it is more C-shaped than the lateral, which displays a more marked curve and approximates a complete circle. The anterior and posterior ends of the medial meniscus are attached to the anterior and posterior intercondylar areas of the articular aspect of the tibia, while the transverse genicular ligament joins the anterior ends of the two menisci. The capsule attaches the menisci to the underlying tibia. In contrast to the lateral meniscus the medial is firmly anchored on its peripheral margin to the deep portion of the tibial collateral ligament and is therefore less mobile than its counterpart.

The same force that caused the injury to the two ligaments also produced the longitudinal tear in the attachment of the medial meniscus to the inner layer of the tibial collateral ligament and displaced the meniscus toward the interior of the joint. Are injuries of the medial meniscus more common than of the lateral, and if so, what is the cause of the difference in frequency? The medial meniscus is injured about seven times more commonly than the lateral. The difference is explained by the firm anchorage of the medial meniscus to the tibial collateral ligament in contrast to the slight mobility of the lateral which seems to assure its escape from damage. Another reason is that the frequency of various sports, such as football, baseball, and skiing, causes an abduction and lateral rotation strain on the flexed knee. What clinical sign in our case indicates possible injury to the medial meniscus? The marked restriction of extension of the knee joint is an indication of displacement of the fibrocartilage toward the center of the joint. In this position the meniscus offers an impediment to passive extension.

The rationale of removal of the injured meniscus lies in the fact that, since it is essentially avascular, traumatic defects do not repair themselves. Occasionally regeneration of a meniscus after removal is reported.

41 Anterior Tibial Syndrome

At the beginning of the football season a 20-year-old college student participated in strenuous field practice extending through the whole afternoon. Later in the evening he experienced severe pain over the anterolateral aspect of his right leg, radiating down toward the ankle. The next afternoon he went back to the field and continued to play, but the pain in his right leg became so severe that he had to limp off the field. The pain persisted throughout the night and the next morning he consulted a physician.

EXAMINATION

On examination there is reddening and swelling over the anterolateral aspect of his right leg. On palpation this area is extremely tender, it feels hard and warmer than other parts of the leg. The hardening extends from two inches below the tibial tuberosity to the junction of the middle and lower thirds of the leg and seems to correspond to the belly of the tibialis anterior muscle. Dorsiflexion of foot and toes is severely limited. The pulses in the anterior tibial and dorsalis pedis arteries are present. His body temperature is slightly elevated.

THERAPY AND FURTHER COURSE

The patient is hospitalized and his leg is immobilized by splinting; moist packs are applied to it. Since there is no improvement within the next twenty-four hours, the fascia over the anterolateral aspect of the leg is incised under general anesthesia. The muscles in the anterior compartment of the leg show some grayish-brown discoloration and seem rather hard to the touch. Muscle biopsies are taken from the discolored areas for microscopic studies which show signs of degeneration and necrosis (cell death) in the muscle fibers. The fascia is left wide open, but the skin over it is partially closed.

In the next few days there is discharge of necrotic material from the site of incision, but the pain and fever subside. During the following weeks exudation from the wound gradually stops and the wound closes. Dorsiflexion of the foot and toes continue to be restricted, but the patient is able to walk and is discharged.

DIAGNOSIS

We are dealing with a disease that has come to be known by the name "anterior tibial syndrome."

DISCUSSION

The condition is caused by an acute impairment of the intramuscular circulation in the muscles of the anterior compartment of the leg. It is assumed that heavy exercise, particularly in an individual who is not conditioned, causes a swelling of the musculature, perhaps also some tearing of muscle fibers and small hemorrhages inside the muscles. This increase in bulk compresses the smaller vessels within the muscle bellies which in turn leads to degeneration and necrosis of muscle fibers. Identify the muscles in the anterior compartment of the leg. The tibialis anterior is particularly affected, and the extensor hallucis longus is affected to a greater extent and more commonly than the extensor digitorum longus and peroneus tertius. What in the configuration of the anterior compartment makes this region particularly liable to increase in intracompartmental pressure? Keep in mind that this compartment is

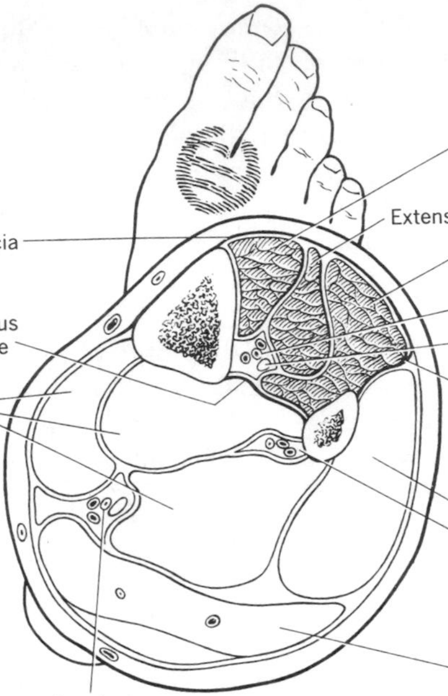

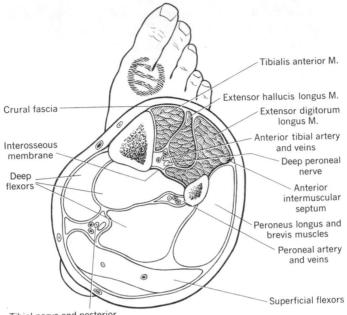

Figure 1 shows a cross-section through the right leg at junction of intermediate and lower thirds of leg. Notice muscles, nerve and blood vessels in closed anterior compartment.

Also notice area of sensory loss on dorsum of foot in paralysis of deep peroneal nerve.

bounded by rigid or semi-rigid walls, formed by the tibia, fibula, interosseous membrane, crural fascia, and anterior intermuscular septum (Fig. 1). Remember that the latter septum separates the anterior from the lateral compartment which contains the peroneous longus and brevis muscles.

Involvement of the deep peroneal nerve

The major nerve and blood vessels in the compartment may also be affected by the elevation in pressure. Identify them. The deep peroneal nerve and the anterior tibial vessels are important structures in the compartment. How would you test for involvement of the deep peroneal nerve, keeping in mind that dorsiflexion of foot and toes may be severely interfered with by anoxia (lack of oxygen) of the muscles in the compartment, and that loss of muscle action therefore does not necessarily imply nerve involvement? What muscle supplied by the deep peroneal nerve lies outside the compressed compartment, the paralysis of which could be taken as an indication of direct nerve involvement? The extensor digitorum brevis on the dorsum of the foot lies outside the anterior compartment and consequently beyond the site of direct attack by pressure, but is also supplied by the deep peroneal nerve. Its paralysis would prove that the compression involves the deep peroneal nerve within the compartment. Deficiencies in the sensory supply of the skin would also demonstrate that the deep peroneal nerve is directly affected. What area of the skin would you test for sensory loss? The adjacent sites of the first and second toes receive their sensory supply from the deep peroneal nerve (Fig. 1).

Arterial involvement

The presence of arterial pulse in the anterior tibial and dorsalis pedis artery seems to prove patency of the main stem, although, occasionally, a well-established collateral circulation in the lower part of the leg by means of branches from the arteries in the posterior compartment may simulate patency in a vessel blocked higher up. What vessel in the posterior compartment would particularly contribute to such collateral circulation? The peroneal artery has an important perforating branch that anastomoses with distal branches of the anterior tibial and with the dorsalis pedis artery.

The pulses of the foot

Where do you feel the pulse of the anterior tibial artery? Its pulse is best taken where it becomes superficial just above the level of the ankle joint midway between the malleoli. Where would you palpate the pulse of the dorsalis pedis artery? Remember that this artery is directed across the dorsum of the foot to the proximal end of the first intermetatarsal space. Here it lies on the skeleton of the foot just lateral to the tendon of the extensor hallucis longus. The pulse of the posterior tibial artery should be felt halfway between the posterior margin of the medial malleolus and the medial border of the tendo calcaneus (Achillis) with the foot dorsiflexed and inverted.

The variations in susceptibility of the three main muscles of the anterior compartment to impaired circulation can be explained by differences in the development of the intramuscular arterial anastomoses. Another explanation, frequently offered, is the fact that the anterior tibial muscle has its sole supply from the anterior tibial artery, the less involved extensor hallucis longus receives additional blood from the perforating branch of the peroneal artery, while the extensor digitorum longus obtains its supply from the three major arteries of the leg, including the posterior tibial by way of perforating branches. This latter explanation of the preferential involvement of the anterior tibial muscle presupposes interference with blood flow in the main stem of the anterior tibial artery by elevation of pressure inside the compartment, before its branches enter the musculature. While this occurs, presence of pulsatory excursions in the anterior tibial artery distally and in its continuation, the dorsis pedis artery, as was found in our case, makes this event improbable.

42 Flat Foot

A 33-year-old chef is referred to the Orthopedic Clinic by his family physician because he complains of pain in his feet when standing or walking which worsens as the day progresses. The pain radiates up his legs and into his back. When he comes home, his feet burn and are swollen. In the last few months the pain has increased and is most marked on the medial and plantar sides of his feet. His wife tells him that he "waddles" with his feet turned out in a kind of duck-walk.

EXAMINATION

The patient is an obese man of medium height who on questioning concedes that in the last few years he has gained approximately fifty pounds. On examination the patient is asked to stand on his bare feet with his toes pointing forward and his feet parallel and approximately 4 inches apart. Inspection of his feet from in front and back shows on both sides disappearance of the medial portion of the longitudinal arch which appears completely flattened (Fig. 1). Both feet are everted so that a plumbline dropped from the center of the patella misses the foot entirely, while in the normal condition it strikes the foot between the first and second metatarsal bones (Fig. 2).

The patient is then asked to walk which he does in a clumsy, "Chaplinesque" manner by raising the entire foot at one time instead of rolling it off the ground. On palpation there is

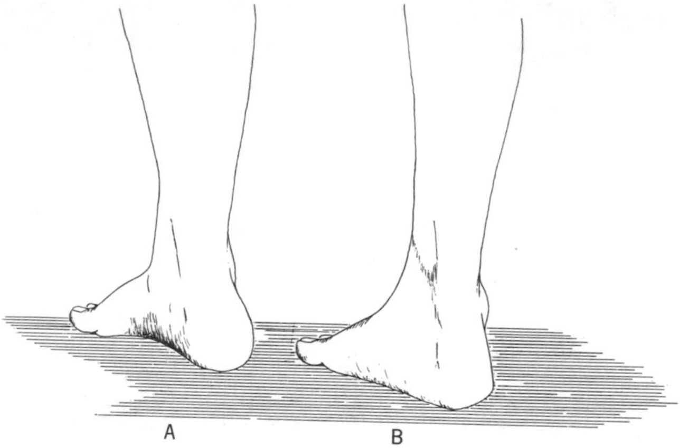

Figure 1. A. Posteromedial view of a normal foot. Notice the longitudinal arch on the medial side of the foot. B. Posteromedial view of a flatfoot. Notice the absence of the longitudinal arch.

tenderness and prominence on the medial plantar side of the foot over the area of the navicular and the head of the talus. By having the patient lie down on a couch and thus removing the body weight from his feet, the longitudinal arch assumes its normal curvature. The movement of the feet are tested in plantar and dorsal flexion, inversion and eversion. Prints of his feet, while weight-bearing, confirm the diagnosis of flatfeet by leaving an imprint of the entire sole on the paper. Finally, inspection of the patient's shoes shows the inner border on the soles and heels worn down to a greater extent than the outer side of the shoes.

DIAGNOSIS

Chronic footstrain due to flatfoot (Pes planus).

THERAPY AND FURTHER COURSE

Conservative (nonsurgical) treatment of this condition aims to relieve the ligaments of the foot of tension and stretching, to

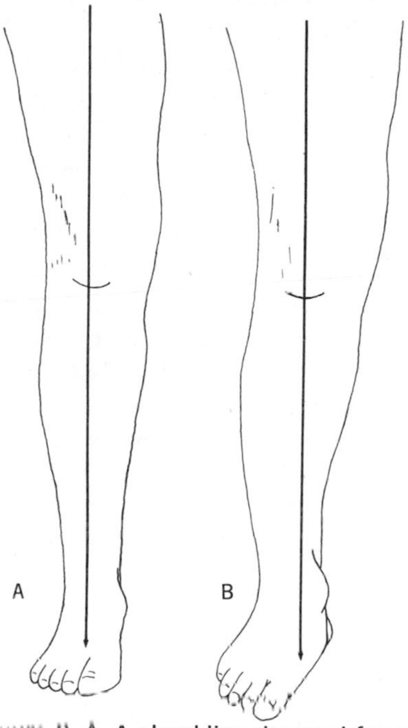

Figure 2. A. A plumbline dropped from the center of the patella strikes the normal foot at a point between the first and second metatarsal. B. In this flatfoot, the same plumbline misses the foot entirely due to pronation of the foot (eversion or valgus deformity).

transfer the weight of the body to the lateral side of the foot, and to strengthen the invertors and plantar flexors, which support the longitudinal arch under stress and in motion. From a cast of the patient's feet an aluminum arch support is shaped, which is sufficiently curved on the medial side to shift the weight of the body to the outer side of the foot. The patient is advised to take hot foot baths, the temperature being raised to the point of tolerance, and begin with massage and passive exercises in the bath, after the acute pain has subsided. These should consist of dorsi- and plantar flexion and should include the toes. They are done at first with the patient sitting down to relieve the feet from weight-bearing. In order to strengthen his invertors, the patient is instructed to invert his feet against increasing resistance offered by his own hand. He also is advised to walk by rolling his feet off the ground from heel to toes. When standing, his feet should be parallel, not turned outward and should be about ten inches apart. He is strongly urged to lose fifty pounds of weight and a diet is recommended. The patient is seen at regular intervals and is given whirlpool baths, manipulations, and massage in the Physical Therapy Department. He volunteers the information that his pain has almost subsided and that his feet have become relatively comfortable. He continues with his foot baths and exercises at home. He has lost thirty pounds of weight and is advised to continue his weight loss and exercises. After six months, a slight adjustment is made in his arch support. He has lost another twenty-five pounds and is now practically asymptomatic.

DISCUSSION

The infirmity that we are dealing with in this case is one of the most common ailments of civilized mankind. It has been estimated that approximately 80 per cent of the population have at one time or other foot trouble of this nature. Another often quoted figure is that among Selective Service subjects, 14 per cent are found to have defective arches. Many of these cases are never seen by a physician but by a chiropodist or podiatrist. However, a sufficient number will consult their family physician, who should be well versed in the diagnosis and treatment of foot ailments. Familiarity with the pathology, diagnosis, and therapy of this often quite disabling affliction requires a detailed knowledge of the underlying anatomy.

Motions of the tarsus; joints, muscles, and nerves concerned

The following terms are used to describe movements of the proximal portion of the foot below the ankle: adduction and abduction, inversion and eversion, and supination and pronation. Try to define these terms. In order to understand the following discussion of the underlying anatomy, the reader is advised to supply himself with an articulated skeleton of the foot or, lacking this, with anatomical atlas figures. Adduction and abduction refer to movement of the foot around a vertical axis through the leg. In inversion and eversion rotation of the foot takes place around an oblique axis that passes from the lateral side of the heel forward, upward, and medially through the neck of the talus. Inversion is the movement whereby the medial margin of the foot is elevated and the dorsum of the foot turned laterally. If inversion is done with both feet at the same time, the soles of the feet face each other. The opposite movement is called eversion. Due to the obliquity of the axis, inversion is combined with adduction of the forefoot and eversion with abduction. The term inversion and supination are often used interchangeably as are eversion and pronation. In what joints do these complex movements take place? The main articulation involved is the talocalcaneonavicular joint, which is a synovial joint of the ball and socket variety. The head of the talus is the ball and is received by the concavity of the posterior surface of the navicular and the anterior and middle articular facets of the calcaneus, the latter belonging to the sustentaculum tali, a shelf, palpable one inch below the medial malleolus. The socket of this joint is completed by the plantar calcaneonavicular (spring) ligament, which is fibrocartilaginous and extends from the sustentaculum tali to the inferior aspect of the navicular. Two other joints concerned in the motions of the tarsus are the calcaneocuboid articulation between the anterior surface of the calcaneus and the posterior surface of the cuboid and the subtalar joint between a facet on the posterior-inferior aspect of the talus and the posterior facet on the superior aspect of the calcaneus. The term "mid-tarsal" joint is frequently used by clinicians and refers to the talonavicular part of the talocalcaneonavicular joint and the calcaneocuboid joint, the latter having a separate synovial cavity. This joint is also the site of a now obsolete surgical disarticulation of the foot, which left only the talus and calcaneus behind and which was introduced in the early part of the 19th century by the French surgeon, Francois Chopart. The joint is, therefore, often referred to as "Chopart's joint." The ability to invert or evert (supinate or pronate) the foot should be appreciated because these motions allow the foot to adjust to sideways sloping surfaces. If inversion or eversion is lost, the patient is severely handicapped in walking over rough ground.

The muscles responsible for these motions are the tibialis anterior and posterior for inversion and adduction and the peronei for eversion and abduction. What nerves supply these muscles? The important motor nerves are the deep peroneal for the tibialis anterior and peroneus tertius, the tibialis nerve for the tibialis posterior, and the superficial peroneal nerve for the supply of the peroneus longus and brevis. Either of these nerves or a combination are frequently involved in poliomyelitis with resulting severe gait disturbances.

The longitudinal arch of the foot

This arch, which comprises the tarsus and metatarsus, consists of inner (medial) and outer (lateral) portions. Both of these share a common posterior pillar, i.e. the tuberosity of the calcaneus. The medial component of the arch is formed, in addition to the calcaneus, by the talus, the navicular, the three cuneiforms, and the medial three metatarsals as the anterior pillar. The outer part of the longitudinal arch is composed of the calcaneus, the cuboid, and the lateral two metatarsals. The medial side of the longitudinal arch curves higher than the lateral, which almost rests on the ground. The talus is the keystone of the arch and receives the body weight which is then distributed to both components of the arch. The weight of the body, therefore, is transferred to the calcaneus and the heads of the five metatarsals, with the first metatarsal bearing more of the weight than the others. However, it should be realized that the arch is not rigid, as it would be if it were made up of one solid curved bone. As the weight of the body shifts in standing, walking, jumping, running, and bearing of burdens, the weight distribution to individual bones also changes. This requires a supple, resilient construction of the foot. Such a demand is ideally fulfilled by a structure made up of multiple components, the small bones of the foot, which assume a curved configuration. These bones are held together by ligaments, tendons, and muscles allowing for continuous alterations in the relationship of the bones.

Supports of the longitudinal arch

As stated, the arched shape of the foot is due to the configuration of the bones, with the individual members of the structure supporting each other. Thus, the sustentaculum tali, which is a process of the calcaneus, buttresses the head of the talus, (sustentaculum [Latin] means prop or support), but the bones alone are not capable of maintaining the stability of the arch. In spite of a large number of investigations, the mechanism of support of the arch is still controversial. One group of investigators contends that the arch is maintained by active contraction of the muscles traversing the foot; another group assigns this task to the ligaments of the foot; and a third group holds that a combination of both of these structures is responsible. In the past, most anatomists have asserted that muscles are indispensable to the maintenance of the longitudinal arch and that ligaments alone are insufficient for support of the arch. Recent evidence, however, based on electromyographic studies, allows the conclusion that in normal quiet standing the arch is maintained by ligamentous structures without assistance from muscles which show only slight intermittent activity when minor shifts in balance occur. Thus, the first line of defense against physical stress in the standing position are the ligaments (Basmajian). Identify the ligaments that maintain the arch in the standing-at-ease posture. The most important is the plantar aponeurosis which, like a tie-beam, extends between the anterior and posterior pillars of the arch, i.e. the heads of the metatarsals and the tuberosity of the calcaneus. Of almost equal importance is the plantar calcaneonavicular (spring) ligament, which directly supports the head of the talus, the summit of the arch. It is a broad, thick, powerful fibrocartilaginous ligament whose attachments have been listed before. It blends on its outside with the capsule of the plantar calcaneonavicular joint and except where it is cartilaginous, is lined by synovia. Other ligaments that help to maintain the arch and resist its flattening are the long and short plantar ligaments in the sole of the foot and the interosseous ligaments between individual tarsal bones but particularly between talus and calcaneus. They truly keep the bones together and prevent them from spreading or splaying. What is the role of the muscles passing through the foot in maintaining the arch? In the face of contradictory and conflicting statements in the literature, Basmajian, on the basis of experiments with needle electrodes inserted into the muscles, concluded that the tibialis anterior, tibialis posterior, and peroneus longus, as well as the short intrinsic muscles of the foot, play no important role in the normal static support of the longitudinal arch. Most of these muscles show inactivity during standing in a relaxed position. They enter the picture only when the foot is exposed to heavy loads or when standing on tiptoe. They also keep the foot balanced around its oblique anteroposterior axis when, due to slight changes in posture, the weight on the foot shifts. However, in walking, particularly in the initiation of the gait, the muscles are strongly activated.

Causes and mechanism of flatfoot

If due to hereditary causes, obesity, or prolonged periods of standing, a weakening of the ligaments occurs, the talus, which is the summit of the medial arch, sags under the force of the superimposed weight of the body and rolls off the calcaneus in a downward and medial direction. In this position it exerts undue pressure on the spring ligament and stretching of this and the previously identified plantar ligaments occurs. The result is a medially flattened arch with prominence of the talus on the medial aspect of the foot and convexity of its inner margin. The foot assumes an eversion or valgus position (Fig. 1). Which of these causes of flatfoot apply to our patient? He has gained a great deal of weight. His occupation as chef requires long periods of standing without exercise of the foot muscles. Occupations such as baker, chef, traffic policeman, operating room nurse, and dentist are particularly liable to foot-strain and flattening of the longitudinal arch. As has been mentioned in our case history, a plumbline dropped from the center of the patella misses the foot entirely. This is due to eversion and abduction of the foot (Fig. 2). Also noted was the greater wearing down of the shoes on the inner side of the soles and heels. Other causes of flatfoot are weakening and relaxation of the ligaments and atrophy of the supporting muscles due to prolonged bed-confinement in chronic illness or extended plaster immobilization of the foot for traumatic or orthopedic disorders.

A congenitally shortened Achilles tendon, or uncounter-balanced action of the peroneal muscles changes the line of gravity and puts the foot in a position of pronation (Pes valgus), thus increasing the stress on the weight sustaining ligaments.

In this discussion of the causes of flatfoot, it should be clearly understood that such a condition cannot be equated with painful feet or chronic foot-strain. Many flatfeet function normally and never give rise to clinical symptoms. It also has to be realized that the condition of flatfoot is often erroneously diagnosed in infancy or early childhood where the longitudinal arch is obscured by a pad of fat, which fills the sole of the foot. Later as the child grows, much of the fat disappears and the arch becomes demonstrable.

Muscle activity in maintaining the stance in flatfoot

We may ask ourselves to what extent the long and short muscles of the foot are called upon for support after the ligaments have weakened. Preliminary findings of Basmajian and coworkers seem to indicate that the tibialis anterior and posterior, the peroneus longus, and certain short muscles in the sole are activated in disorders of the foot that lead to imbalance of the arch. While the ligaments of the foot are the first line of defense in maintaining the arch, extrinsic and intrinsic muscles are needed for additional support in flatfoot. These muscles are also called upon to support the arch in the so-called military stance. Here with the toes turned outward and the heels in apposition, the body weight is imposed on the inner side of the foot. The talus rolls downward and medially off the calcaneus, causing a bulge along the inner border of the foot. Thus by putting the foot in the pronated (valgus) position, the military posture exposes the medial side of the arch to great strain and may eventually lead to a weak and painful flatfoot.

Pain in flatfoot

The primary pain of flatfoot is due to stretching of the ligaments, mainly the spring and plantar ligaments, occasionally also the deltoid ligament on the medial side of the ankle joint. When the muscles are charged with the task of maintaining the longitudinal arch, even when standing at ease, they fatigue and respond to the strain with pain. If the condition remains uncorrected, the construction of the foot is altered by the changing relationship of the bones to each other. In that case, other muscles, such as the calf muscles, may become involved and painful. Undue stretching of the ligaments of the knee joint and even of the spinal column may cause pain in these areas. An aching back is not uncommon in chronic footstrain. Painful calluses may develop over pressure points on bony prominences of the foot which normally do not touch the ground. If the footstrain develops rapidly, as in prolonged illness, fine tears of the ligaments, which can be observed under the microscope, explain the pain and tenderness on pressure.